THE
H
WORD

The diagnostic studies to evaluate symptoms,
alternatives in treatment,
and coping with the aftereffects of hysterectomy.

Nora W. Coffey
and
Rick Schweikert

*Give this book
to a gynecologist.*

Table of Contents

THE

H

WORD

ONE

"Things like this don't happen to women like me."

The Protest & Play Year—Nora W. Coffey

This is a book about the uterus and the ovaries. What they are, where they're located, and their many important life-long functions. The common reasons women are told they need treatment, including surgery, as well as alternatives in treatment and the ways that hysterectomy (removal of the uterus) and oophorectomy (removal of the ovaries, castration) impacts a woman's body, her health, and every aspect of her life.

Until recently, the H word was rarely discussed openly outside a gynecologist's office. Only 3/10^{ths} of one percent of the women who contact the Hysterectomy Educational Resources and Services Foundation (HERS)—three out of every thousand hysterectomized women—say they were educated prior to surgery about the consequences of removing this powerful muscle.

Most of us know women who say they're "just fine" after the surgery, and the reasons are so complex it takes a book like this to understand why. The anatomical facts of hysterectomy and castration are universal and should be made public so women are aware of their far-reaching consequences before they're told to sign a hysterectomy consent form.

The last 25 years of my life have been dedicated to educating women about their female organs, so when a doctor tells them they need a hysterectomy they'll know what questions to ask—and the answers to those questions—to evaluate the doctor's recommendation. HERS is a highly successful model for hysterectomy, providing information required for "informed consent" to millions of people worldwide and counseling to more than 850,000 women. About half of those women call HERS searching for information prior to surgery, and the other half are searching for answers after the surgery. A vast majority of the women who call HERS learn about conservative treatments, including no treatment, and they don't undergo the surgery.

And still, doctors conduct unnecessary hysterectomy and castration every minute of every hour of every day. After 25 years, I continued exploring ways to solve the lack of informed consent that is at the heart of this problem.

I was on my way from Philadelphia to Brooklyn to visit my son and daughter-in-law for Thanksgiving. The HERS Foundation's production of Rick Schweikert's play *un becoming* was set to open in conjunction with our 23rd annual Hysterectomy Conference in New York.[1] Planning the conference while premiering the play Off Broadway was a major undertaking. I was so restless, it took driving up the New Jersey turnpike alone with my thoughts to put things into perspective.

I had met Rick only a year before, in December of 2002. It seemed like an incidental meeting at the time. After briefly addressing a real estate concern, I sensed there was much more to this intense, kind man than real estate development.

He asked me what I "do" in Philadelphia. I told him I was the founder and president of the HERS Foundation. When the word "hysterectomy" came up, I saw in his eyes the first flicker of curiosity. He wanted to know why this surgery required an organization to educate the public about it. Then he asked another question. And another. For six hours he asked and I responded.

---

[1] http://unbecomingplay.com.

He didn't flinch. He was incredulous, even shocked, but he wanted to know everything.

In the months following that meeting, we exchanged hundreds of emails, spoke on the phone for hours at a time, and we spent entire days and evenings together talking about hysterectomy when he visited me in Philadelphia. I answered his questions and sometimes told him things he didn't want to hear. With sensitivity and grace, he didn't turn away when I spoke about my own experiences. For the first time since I was hysterectomized and castrated, I felt safe journeying back in time.

For years, my days were spent counseling many thousands of women—listening and sometimes validating their experiences by telling them the exterior of my own. But quite unexpectedly, by telling Rick the most private details of my experiences, I began to relive the horror of it all in real time—the day a gynecologist changed my body and my life forever.

As if peeling off layers of my own skin, images and details that were deliberately walled off decades before came crashing into the present. I found myself transported back to the day I arrived at the hospital. I had been admitted because of abdominal pains, and stayed there a few days before the doctor finally convinced me I should let him perform exploratory surgery to remove an ovarian mass. The purpose of the surgery, I was told, was to determine if the ovarian mass was cancerous. A nurse sedated me shortly before an orderly transferred me from a bed to a gurney. I felt a sense of foreboding as I was wheeled from my hospital room to the elevator. When the doors closed, I felt like I was suffocating, like something catastrophic was about to happen. So each time someone walked by, I said, "Excuse me, I need to speak with

Dr. Giuntoli." I yelled out to them as they walked away, "I changed my mind about the surgery," but no one stopped.

Even as I protested, I was transferred from the gurney to the operating table. I resisted as they strapped down my 90-pound, 5-foot frame. "Let me up!" I said, "I changed my mind." I pulled at the straps while one person held my arms against my side and the other tightened the straps around me. No one said anything or seemed to hear me. I was just one of many women no one would bother to hear.

The anesthesiologist taped my arm to a board. He reassured me everything was going to be okay. He ignored my pleas to let me get up. I was struggling to free myself when I felt the needle go into my arm. I kept repeating, "Stop. I changed my mind. Stop!" even as I went under.

Although we had only agreed to conservative surgery, unless there was cancer of the ovary, when I woke up I discovered that Giuntoli had hysterectomized and castrated me without my informed consent. And there was no cancer.

As I recounted all of this to Rick, images of intricate details flooded my consciousness. I remembered the crack in the corner of the dirty green plaster operating room wall. The time frozen on the clock. The sudden terror of realizing that something irreversible was about to be done to my body.

Suddenly, I was laid bare again. I wasn't prepared for what would come from telling a relative stranger things I had kept to myself for so long. Throughout the next few months, like an endless loop it played and replayed over and over again. I couldn't sleep, and even when I could, I woke up screaming with torrents of tears.

And then one day Rick called to say he was writing a play about hysterectomy. As he casually described a scene he was working on, I thought, "How dare he." Someone else writing about my most personal and intimate thoughts without my consent? Even then he didn't turn away from my anger and anguish. He quietly kept writing.

When he asked me what I thought about him coming to Philadelphia to read the first draft of his play to me, I hesitated. I wasn't sure I'd be able to cope with it. Could anyone possibly put into words this confusing, harsh reality? But he persevered. As he read his then untitled play to me, the tears flowed again, this time with awe for the beauty of his writing and the depth of his understanding.

He then took his play into a series of workshops in New York. He and the cast worked and reworked every scene. He called several times a day with updates.

At the end of each day of counseling, I knew there were a few more women out there who would avoid unnecessary surgeries because they received information from HERS. It was too little too late, however, for 621,000 other women in this country each year—more than 22 million hysterectomized women alive in America today.[2] I'm haunted daily by the feeling that I'm not doing enough, that I could do more.

un becoming was a success. I knew the play would make its mark. It would alert people in a unique and powerful way. With the end of the run of the play in sight, I began to think about what

[2] 621,000 is a 10-year average from 1996 to 2005, from the Centers for Disease Control and Prevention (CDC), National Center for Health Statistics (NCHS). 22 million is an estimate by the HERS Foundation, based on NCHS inpatient hospital discharge data.

would come next. I wanted the next step in our efforts to educate the public to build on that expanding awareness about hysterectomy—something very public, very open.

On that drive from Philadelphia to Brooklyn for Thanksgiving dinner, I began making plans for a nationwide, yearlong protest. By the time I arrived at my son's house, a rough outline of the entire protest year was fully formed. I don't carry a tape recorder, so I called my voice mail and dictated all the whats, whens, wheres, and hows. A protest...in each state...every week...for an entire year.

I thought about the hundreds of thousands of women I had counseled throughout the last 25 years in every corner of the country. The protest would be a way for them to take back some of the power that had been taken from them. It would be a collective effort, but I envisioned it as an individual experience for each woman in her own hometown, in front of the hospital where a doctor had taken her sex organs from her. It seemed right to protest where the crime was done. If we protested at the hospitals themselves, the doctors, administrators, and assistants could still look away from us, but they couldn't avoid us. They would know that we know what they're doing to women. That we were going to make it public all across the country.

Later, Rick added notes to my plans. We talked about the play being part of it and began referring to it as the Protest & Play year. "There's no reason we can't have the play in all these cities," Rick said. But we realized that taking the New York cast to 51 cities in 51 weeks would be financially and logistically impossible. So he suggested readings of the play, as opposed to full productions. "Readings will be easy," he said.

I was skeptical. And, in fact, producing all those readings with a different cast in each city would prove to be a daunting task. Rick wouldn't be able to schedule some of them until a few weeks prior to arriving there. He'd have to educate the actors quickly from the ground up, just as I had to educate him and he educated the cast in New York. He'd most likely have to work with actors who'd resist this education. Most of them would know someone who'd been hysterectomized. Some of the actors would be doctors, nurses, or hysterectomized women themselves. Some theater companies would be receptive to the central message, others wouldn't. He'd have to change the dogmatic minds of actors and directors who might insist on an incorrect or even damaging perception of hysterectomy.

It seemed that the most logical place to start was in Birmingham, Alabama, the heart of the Civil Rights Movement. Once that decision was made, our main concern was spending the winter months in the South and the summer months in the North. Rick highlighted the protests we could lead together and was disappointed to discover he could only attend about half of them. I'd be leading the other half alone.

Neither of us fully realized what we were in for. We were both veteran protestors in support of many civil rights issues, but this protest would be different. It would be more political, more radical, and more personal. The majority of the women I had counseled had never taken part in a protest.

Rick was worn out from putting the play together in New York. I was exhausted from traveling back and forth between New York and keeping HERS running smoothly in Philadelphia. But we didn't hesitate. We both said, "Let's do it."

TWO

What's a uterus worth?

Birmingham, Alabama: Rick Schweikert

Debra, our Alabama organizer, suggested that we meet for breakfast at the diner where she worked. For the protesters there was a sense of relief to be in the company of other women who could talk openly about hysterectomy. As they came through the door of the diner, it was as if they'd been wandering around lost and suddenly found a portal back to the familiar, like foreigners who happened to stumble into the one restaurant where everyone spoke their language. Thoughts and feelings bottled up inside of them suddenly flowed freely.

Some arrived from distant places, others from just a few miles away. "When was your hysterectomy?" they asked each other. Some answered with not just the year, but the month, the day, and even the hour and minute of the day they were hysterectomized.

A sense of awe at the enormity of what we were embarking on prevailed over introductions each time another protestor arrived. Nora greeted each protestor and introduced them to me. She had counseled most of these women on the phone, but this was the first time Nora had met most of them in person.

I checked my satchel again to make sure I had the permit from the City of Birmingham for our public demonstration. The waitress gracefully danced between the tables, bending an ear to drop in on our conversations.

Somehow, somewhere along the way, it would become commonplace to have a waiter, bartender, or the person at the next table bending an ear to eavesdrop in on us. As soon as the H word was spoken, we generally had the attention of everyone around us, whether we wanted it or not. But it took a while for me to get comfortable talking about it in public. At some point I'd stop caring if anyone overheard. We had a right and a responsibility to speak openly about what the medical industrial establishment was doing to women. If anyone was offended, then maybe being offended was an appropriate response.

The need for a demonstration probably wasn't self-evident to the regulars there in the diner. They probably hadn't ever met someone like Nora. Nor were they likely to have read testimony from women spanning generations, or Congressional hearings confirming that hysterectomy permanently damages women and is rarely medically warranted.[3] The hysterectomy rate in the South is 50% higher than it is in the Northeast,[4] though, so it's very likely that the people in that diner knew someone whose life had been altered by the surgery. Even if that person didn't talk openly about it with them.

Some people are quick to scold other cultures and societies for intentional injuries such as female genital mutilation, while turning a deaf ear to what's being done to women right here in the U.S. Uninformed and misinformed consent is unwanted touching. Like rape, unwanted touching is a crime. And as we demonstrate throughout this book, almost none of the 621,000 hysterectomies performed each year on American women are consented, because

---

[3] A Congressional hearing on unnecessary surgery in 1976 found that hysterectomies for cancer prevention or sterilization were unjustified. The second Congressional hearing in 1993 concluded that, "90 percent are performed more out of folklore and tradition than proven effectiveness."

[4] Centers for Disease Control and Prevention (CDC), National Center for Health Statistics (NCHS).

women are denied the information required to provide *informed* consent. Women only learn about the consequences of hysterectomy by experiencing the irreversible, permanent aftermath. We scoff at societies where women wear *niqab* or *burqa* veils that cover their faces, but we avert our eyes from what's being done to our own mothers, daughters, sisters, and friends.

"I've never spoken with anyone about this except Nora," one woman said. "I never thought I'd see the day I'd be protesting in front of a hospital." Overcome by hearing these words from her own mouth in public, tears filled her eyes. Nora went to her side. Others in the diner continued looking at us curiously. A spoon slowly turned inside a cup of coffee and then clinked three times on the side of the cup. The line cook flipped sausages and hash-browns on a sizzling grill. A large man periodically peeked over the Sports Section of the newspaper at us.

"It's important to be precise about the language," Nora said. "I never say I *had* a hysterectomy. It's something that was done *to* me. It's not something I chose like ordering from a menu."

The decision to remove their female organs was made while many of these women were anesthetized. And for all of them it was unconsented.

The woman who was crying said, "My doctor just laughed at me. She said, 'Oh, that's all in your head.' I trusted her because she's a woman, but she bullied me in a way I don't think any male doctor could have." The other women nodded their heads, knowingly.

Protest permits were being arranged in 51 cities. We wrote press releases and listed the protests and readings of *un becoming* on events calendars. Protest signs and educational materials had been printed. A complex schedule of what was to be sent where ensured that signs and materials would await organizers at each location throughout the year. As we gathered in Birmingham those materials were beginning to zigzag across the country. Airline tickets, hotel accommodations, and car rental reservations had been booked. The organizers were given *The Right To Protest: The Basic ACLU Guide to Free Expression.*[5] We discussed what to do and what not to do while we drove single-file downtown to the University of Alabama-Birmingham Medical Center.

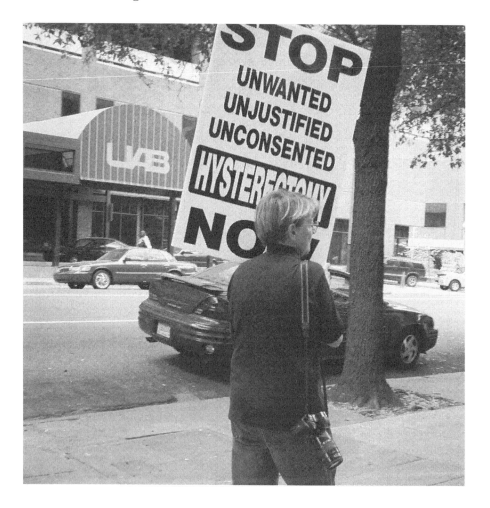

---

[5] Gora, Goldberger, Stern, and Halperin, *The Right To Protest: The Basic ACLU Guide to Free Expression*, Southern Illinois University Press, 1991.

We stood on the sidewalk in front of the main entrance to the hospital near a row of newspaper vending machines in the massive canyon between the UAB Medical Center buildings. "Shoot," one of the protestors said, "it's like David versus Goliath."

In spite of all the planning, no one knew what to expect. Protestors distributing educational materials would be an unwelcome sight for the hospitals that benefited from hysterectomy profits. The revenue from immediate hospital and doctor charges for medically unwarranted hysterectomies is about $17B/year.[6] The cost to families and communities is incalculable. How much pressure would the doctors and hospital administrators who were profiting from hysterectomy put on local police to deny us our First Amendment right to protest? Plenty. Would we be harassed, intimidated? Yes. Arrested?

Throughout the year Nora would maintain her busy counseling schedule, fielding calls from hotel rooms, rental cars, airports, or while standing at a protest, phone in one hand and a protest sign in the other. By then HERS had counseled more than 850,000 women over a period of 23 years. She would continue that work while taking HERS' mandate to the streets.

The rules were to stay off hospital property and to not obstruct traffic. Without hesitation each protestor took up a sign and began marching back and forth in front of the hospital. A few of the signs read:

---

[6] Based on average costs from recent itemized hospital bills of women counseled by HERS, first published by Rick Schweikert as "12-Minute Video to Save Health Insurance Providers More than $17B/Year," *Health Insurance Underwriter Magazine*, August 2007.

STOP!

HYSTERECTOMY

DAMAGES WOMEN

HYSTERECTOMY:

SURGICAL

VIOLENCE

STOP

CASTRATING WOMEN

NOW

The protests were scheduled to take place 11:00 a.m. to 1:00 p.m. About a half hour before the end of the first day, the Birmingham police arrived to tell us we wouldn't be allowed to continue protesting.

"On what grounds?" Nora asked.

"There was a complaint."

"A complaint about what?" I asked.

"You need a permit to do this."

"I don't remember anything in the First Amendment about a permit," I said. I thought about how in May 1963 Kelly Ingram Park (about a mile away) became the epicenter of the Civil Rights Movement. "But we do have one," I said.

"May I see it?"

Just then more police motorcycles and cars arrived on the scene. A few of them stood with their thumbs in their belts, staring-down the protestors who couldn't have been a less menacing group. The first cop spoke on her cell phone with someone down at the precinct about the permit. I asked the others to continue protesting.

Regardless of the intentions of the person who called the police in the first place, the result was good for us. People were curious about our protest before, but now they were lingering to show their support, saying things like, "What're they here for, this is a free country, isn't it?"

Finally, the cop motioned me back over. She smiled, telling us to stay out of the street, to stay off hospital property, and to not obstruct foot traffic, "Because they will have you arrested," she said.

"They?" I said, as Nora handed her a pamphlet.

That night a staged reading of *un becoming* was hosted by the UAB Women's Studies Program, performed by the Birmingham Park Players. A quote from women's health writer Barbara Seaman was used to promote the readings: "Every woman, man and child should see this play!"

With one rehearsal under their belt, the cast moved the audience in Birmingham as much as the full production did in New York. During the performance, one of the protestors—hysterectomized at only 20 years old—left the reading in tears, comforted by a friend.

At the end of *un becoming* the actor playing Halley delivers a monologue directly to the audience as she steps down off the stage and exits the theater. Her final words are the last lines of the play:

> Every morning I wake up, I look out the window, and I'm amazed that women aren't screaming in the streets. Every life split in two should be an atomic explosion, instead it just results in more...silence. Every story is too unbelievable

to be true. And yet, there's another one every minute of every hour of every day. Something must be done….I'm through watching. This thing must stop. This *thing* must stop!

After one of the first shows in New York, a woman stood up, saying, "I don't know what the rest of you thought about this play, but I just wanted to say that what happened on this stage tonight is exactly what happened to me!" I was out in the lobby and returned to the theater to lead the spontaneous talkback. The cast returned too, to help me take questions. After that, Nora attended every show, and by the time we arrived in Birmingham we were getting comfortable with the talkbacks.

After the Birmingham reading, a young woman sitting alone asked, "Well, if all of this is true, why do women have hysterectomies?"

"Because they've been acculturated to trust doctors," Nora told her. "I can assure you if doctors said, 'Okay, this is what I'm going to do when I operate on you: I'm going to remove your uterus, which is a hormone-responsive reproductive sex organ that supports your bladder and bowel. If you experience uterine orgasm, you'll never experience it again after the surgery. You'll have a loss of feeling in your clitoris, labia, vagina, and nipples, because a spaghetti-like bundle of nerves called the hypogastric plexus must be severed to remove the uterus.' But doctors don't tell women this. They don't tell them that *Te Linde's Operative Gynecology* says of the hypogastric plexus, 'This latter extension contains the fibers that innervate the vestibular bulbs and clitoris.'[7] And it can't be reattached. They don't tell women your vagina will be shortened,

---

[7] Rock, John A. and Jones, Howard W., *Te Linde's Operative Gynecology*, Lippincott Williams & Wilkins, 7th Edition, 1992.

scarred, and sutured into a closed pocket. And they don't say, 'While I'm there, I'm going to castrate you by removing your ovaries.' You can be sure that if doctors provided women with all the information they need to make informed decisions, that would be the end of unwarranted hysterectomies."

The woman who asked the question became more introspective, her eyebrows knitted as she processed Nora's response. It was an expression we'd become familiar with throughout the year, as people we spoke with slowly "got it."

"What doctors *tell* women they'll experience after the surgery and what women *actually* experience are two totally different things," Nora continued. "Doctors know exactly what they're doing to women because they're the ones holding the scalpel or the laser. But women don't understand what's done to them until it's too late."

The young woman leaned her head into her hands, elbows on her knees, and looked down at her feet as Nora continued.

"Doctors tell women they won't menstruate anymore and they won't be able to have children, but that's about it. And when women tell doctors about all the problems they're having after the surgery, doctors dismiss them, saying, 'Ah, that's all in your head.' But the losses aren't psychological, they're anatomical and physiological. Sex organs have been removed, and the aftermath is devastating. Women experience a diminished or total loss of sexual feeling, vitality, short-term memory, maternal feeling, an increase in heart disease, osteoporosis, difficulty socializing, and a host of other problems they didn't have before the surgery. They're told it's a routine operation, but there's nothing routine about it."[8]

---

[8] "Adverse Effects Data," HERS Foundation, www.hersfoundation.org/effects.html.

The woman nodded her head "yes" with each point, her face slowly softening from disbelief to understanding. A long silence followed. Someone else started to speak, but the young woman Nora had just addressed said to no one in particular, "That's what happened to my mom."

The room fell silent. There were a lot of silent rooms that year. A mixture of guilt, misunderstanding, and loneliness had suddenly been coaxed from behind closed doors as the facts about what her mother had been living with became clear.

The husband of one of the protestors said, "So, why do doctors do this to women?"

"Greed is part of it," Nora said, "doctors become wealthy performing hysterectomies. As the lawyer and women's health advocate Sybil Shainwald, said, 'Hysterectomy isn't just the bread and butter of gynecology, it's the goldmine.' But it's about more than money…it's about power. Removing the female organs is a powerful thing to do to women."

Sometimes it was difficult finding a good place to stop the talkbacks and thank everyone for coming. As with every performance, a few people hung around as we packed up and headed out the door. The discussion continued out of the building and onto the sidewalk in front of the UAB Arts & Humanities Building.

The next day we were back at the protest site in front of the hospital. The director of the UAB Women's Studies Program joined us.

Patients connected to IV poles reached over the boundary of the hospital property to take pamphlets from us, which they read as they smoked cigarettes on the patio near the main entrance. Employees read them as they sat in the shade eating lunch before returning to work. Some doctors (especially the gynecologists) hurried by, veering away, refusing the materials we handed them. Other doctors and nurses stopped to take the information and speak with us.

"Well sure," one doctor said to me matter-of-factly, "I'm not a gynecologist, so I don't mind telling you they do a lot more of them here than they need to." He shrugged his shoulders as if to say, "Oh well," tapped the pamphlet against the palm of his hand, and returned to his job inside the hospital. A young doctor darted out a side door to catch the protest on videotape, before quickly stepping back inside when we spotted him.

No one from the hospital administration came out to speak with us. Cameras flashed from hospital rooms and balconies, and curious patients pressed their faces to the windows. It was quite a sight for Birmingham where the university, which the Medical Center is a huge revenue-generating component, was at that time more than 3-to-1 the area's number one employer. Another hospital corporation, Baptist Health System, was second.[9]

A doctor in a white coat with a stethoscope around his neck quickly walked by. When I handed him a pamphlet he looked at the sign I was carrying, saying, "That's not true, hysterectomy does not damage women!"

"I'd like to talk with you about it," I replied, practically jogging to keep up with him. But he kept walking like we were in a footrace. "If you're right," I asked, "then why won't you talk with me about it?"

---

[9] "Top 30 Employers," Birmingham Regional Chamber of Commerce, March 2008.

One car after another passed by, the drivers and passengers mouthing the five syllables of a word they may have never seen before in print: "hys-ter-ec-to-my." A few medical staff in their hospital greens or white lab coats flipped us off as they drove away in their sports cars. But most of the people driving by honked and gave us a thumbs-up. African-American women and men were more receptive to us than others. They may not have been surprised to hear that hysterectomy rates for women of color are almost 20% higher than the rest of the female population. [10]

A local television station showed up. A few protestors hid behind their signs, afraid of being seen on the evening news. Others were eager to see their signs on TV.

The police arrived again to tell us to disperse. We told them we wouldn't leave until 1:00 p.m. They asked to see our protest permit again. The same police officer from the day before took a step toward me. Staring blankly at the permit, she agreed that we were peaceful and within our rights, but the hospital was going to make sure they "visited us" every day.

"We have a permit," Nora said, "so who are you protecting?"

"It doesn't matter," I said, "we're glad you're out here flashing your lights—it draws more attention to our protest." But still they waited for us to disperse at 1:00 p.m.

One of the protestors stopped a nurse on her way into the hospital. "I was the picture of health before the surgery," the protestor said to the nurse, "and now I can barely stand on my feet for

[10] Centers for Disease Control and Prevention (CDC), National Center for Health Statistics (NCHS).

twenty minutes at a time." The nurse handed the pamphlet back to her, saying, "No thank you," and marched inside the hospital.

We knew that every person who worked in that hospital benefited from hysterectomy. Their livelihoods depended on keeping the beds full. Like any hotel, an empty bed is lost revenue. Even the cafeteria dishwasher I talked with understood that the hospital was a business first and a place of healing second. When he returned to his job after lunch he shook my hand, saying, "Well, thanks for caring."

The protest continued throughout the week. Most people thanked us for the information we gave them. A few women seemed embarrassed, hurt, or downright angry we were out there when they walked by with their families. Our intention was to inform the public, not expose hysterectomized women and their problems. But how could we do the one without the other?

Some of those women literally ran away from us. "I don't intend to talk about my hysterectomy with you or anyone else!" one woman said to me. I hoped that didn't mean she'd remain silent if this was being done to her daughter and granddaughter.

THREE

The "Mississippi Appendectomy"

Jackson, Mississippi—Nora W. Coffey

In the South, sterilization has been called "the Mississippi appendectomy."[11] The U.S. Department of Health and Human Services reports that 57.1% of women aged 65 and older in Mississippi have undergone a hysterectomy.[12] Nationally, one out of every three women is hysterectomized by the age of 60.[13] In Mississippi, it's one out of every three women over the age of 18. Although it may be routine for the doctors who perform the surgery, its aftermath is anything but routine for the women whose female organs are removed. As one woman from Mississippi said in an email, "As a nation, WE HAVE ONE HELLUVA PROBLEM GOING ON HERE!"

A 30 year-old woman I counseled in Mississippi was glad to hear the protest was coming to Jackson, but she wouldn't be there, she said, "Because my husband won't let me." Another woman—in her 40s—couldn't attend, "Because my parents would never let me do that." A third said finding work in Jackson was so difficult she couldn't attend because she was afraid for her hospital job. A fourth said, "My husband doesn't even know I had the surgery. He

[11] Washington, Harriet A., *Medical Apartheid: The Dark History of Medical Experimentation on Black Americans From Colonial Times to the Present*, Doubleday, 2007.
[12] Hysterectomy Status by State, Race/Ethnicity, and Age, 1996-2000. Behavioral Risk Factor Surveillance System, 2000. Survey data, National Center for Chronic Disease Prevention and Health Promotion, Centers for Disease Control and Prevention, U.S. Department of Health and Human Services.
[13] "The Federal Government Source for Women's Health Information," 2000, *US Department of Health & Human Services*, http://www.womenshealth.gov/faq/hysterectomy.cfm.

thinks I had a miscarriage." And one woman said simply, "I'm not well enough to leave my home."

The Jackson protest odyssey began back in Philadelphia. The Jackson Police Department initially indicated that they would "grant" us a permit to protest in front of the Jackson University Medical Center. Later, when we asked about it, they said they had already issued one, but we didn't receive it in the mail. Then they said the permit hadn't been issued, but they were about to fax it to us. Finally, we were told they'd email it to us. But we received nothing.

The "Doctrine Against Prior Restraints" upholds the right of U.S. citizens to assemble and speak freely without being prevented from doing so because of permit restrictions.[14] Permits amount to prior authorization, which is "particularly harmful to free speech values because it suppresses ideas before they are voiced." On the other hand, the authors warn, "protestors faced with an arbitrary permit denial are obliged to abide by the denial until they can get it overturned... Therefore, ignoring an arbitrary or discriminatory permit denial...may result in a speaker being arrested and prosecuted."

Jackson wouldn't be the last city to require a permit and then fail to issue one, but it was the first. It wasn't my wish or intention to be arrested, but the protest would proceed with or without a permit. Waiting for my connecting flight in North Carolina, I called Officer Jerry Brewster. "I'm on my way to Jackson," I said. "I want you to know that I'll be protesting in front of Wiser Hospital tomorrow morning."

[14] Gora, Goldberger, Stern, and Halperin, *The Right To Protest: The Basic ACLU Guide to Free Expression*, Southern Illinois University Press, 1991.

"But you don't have a permit," Officer Brewster said. "Ma'am, you will not be allowed to protest without a permit."

"We applied for it and were told we'd receive it, but it never came. The protest will take place as scheduled."

He was silent for a moment, and then said, "Ma'am, you're going to come here no matter what, aren't you?"

"Yes."

"Okay," he said, "I'll meet you at 8:30 a.m. in front of the hospital, but under no circumstances are you to start without a permit."

I arrived in Jackson later that day and settled into the hotel, catching up on office work and counseling calls.

The next morning Mary and I met in the hallway to head down for breakfast. The elevator took us to the first floor and stopped, but the doors didn't open. Mary was having a full-blown anxiety attack. Apparently, she was even more claustrophobic than me. I called 911 on my cell phone. A large crowd had gathered, and when the fire department opened the doors they cheered for us as we stepped off the elevator. An auspicious beginning to our day.

At breakfast, a waitress in the hotel restaurant asked why we were in town. She wore her hair in the pin-curl style of the 1950s. I told her about HERS and the protest. In response, and quite matter-of-factly, she said, "Really? Well, all of the women in my family had one. My five sisters, my mother…all of them." And then, after a pause she said, "Me too." As it turned out, we only spoke with a few women in Jackson who weren't pregnant who still had a uterus. I handed her a HERS pamphlet, and she began reading it as she walked away.

In the parking lot I realized I left my camera on the table of the restaurant. When I came through the door our waitress was reading the pamphlet to her co-workers. They stood in a circle, one looking over her shoulder and six or seven others leaning against the booths listening closely. That group huddling together gave us our first inkling of just how much of a hidden problem hysterectomy was in Mississippi. It was an accepted rite of passage.

Mary and I arrived at the Winfred L. Wiser Hospital for Women and Infants at the designated time. Officer Brewster wasn't there, so we parked in front of the main entrance and waited. He finally arrived an hour late, without an apology. "Follow me," he said, "I'll meet you across the street." Clearly his intention was to get us off hospital property.

He led the way to a parking lot. Once there he got out of his squad car and spoke to me through the window. "If you insist on protesting," he said, "you'll have to do so over here across the street from the hospital. You won't be allowed to protest in front. Either way, you'll have to get permission from them."

"Permission from the hospital? Even if we stay on public property."

"Yes."

"Listen," I said, "we intend to exercise our right to protest, and we don't need permission from them. The reason we're here without a permit is because your department didn't provide one."

"But a protest over there simply won't be possible," he said, "and if you do, you'll be breaking the law."

"Well," I said, "I guess you'll have to do what you have to do, and we'll have to do what we have to do." And then after a pause, I said, "Why don't you get inside the car and talk with us."

Much to my surprise, he did just that. He asked some questions about hysterectomy and why we were doing this. We talked for a while, and then he said, "Well, you won't be arrested, but you'd better be careful. There are some people who don't want you out here," he said. He then wished us luck, returned to his car, and he was gone.

We crossed the street to the side with the hospital and handed out a lot of information on a busy eight-lane road. One car after another pulled over after reading our signs.

One woman from a town near Jackson said, "All the women in my church had one." She thought about that a moment, before adding, "And all the women in my town go to my church." This stopped me cold. Whole towns where not one woman still had a uterus? Her words paralyzed me, but they would help carry me through the year. It wouldn't be the last time I'd hear that story. We heard the same thing from a woman in Kansas. Two women with different lives from different parts of the country, bearing witness to identical experiences. Whole towns of women hysterectomized. Undoubtedly, the doctors who did this to them also attended their church.

Another woman who pulled over said she had fibroids. Her fibroids weren't causing her any discomfort, and she had no medical problem, but a doctor told her that hysterectomy was the only treatment option. She ignored the horns blaring behind her as Mary, who's a registered nurse, spoke with her through the window of her car. She was determined to get the information she wasn't getting from her doctor.

In every city I looked for two things: a coffeehouse and a bookstore. Not the chain-store variety, but a good local coffeehouse and an independently owned bookstore. Whether these two needs could be met told me something about the city and the people I'd meet there.

But we couldn't find either in Jackson, despite two long forays through the city. Later I'd be interviewed by Ayana Taylor from the Jackson Free Press in a good local coffeehouse, and Ayana also pointed me in the direction of an independent bookstore.

I had a sign made for the rear window of our rental car that said "Hysterectomy Information 877-750-HERS." I bought bungee cords to attach it to whichever car we might rent along the tour. As we drove around Jackson with the sign strapped to the back window, a car pulled up behind us repeatedly honking its horn while flashing its headlights on and off. It then pulled up alongside us in the lane for the oncoming traffic, and the driver motioned for Mary to pull over. When Mary kept driving, the car veered into our lane. Mary had no choice but to pull over to avoid an accident. When our cars came to a stop, we were surprised when a very non-threatening woman put her window down.

"I saw your sign," she said in a rich southern drawl, "and I've been trying to get your attention. I need to speak with you because I already had one, and I need to know about it."

I handed her one of the pamphlets. After quickly perusing it, she repeatedly thanked us and veered back into the traffic, gravel flying out from under her rear wheels.

Mary returned home after the second day of the protest, but before she left we got a bite to eat at a luncheonette. Nurses and other hospital staff were seated at a long table. Mary had her back to them, but she picked up from the conversation that they all worked at Wiser Hospital, where we were protesting. Mary turned around to speak with them, and they asked us why we were there. We told them about the protest, and one of the women who sat with her back to us chuckled.

"What's so funny about women having their sex organs removed?" I asked. "Do they perform many of them at your hospital?"

The first woman to laugh turned around to make eye contact with me, saying, "I had one, and it was best the thing I ever did." The other nurses jovially backed her up.

"Wow," Mary said, "I can't believe that, because it's the *worst* thing that's ever happened to me. What about your sex life?"

The same woman laughed again, saying, "My sex life is great since the surgery." Again, the other nurses agreed.

"Well, I'm glad you're pleased with the results of having your sex organs removed," I said, "but most women don't consider a loss of uterine orgasm to be an improvement in their sex life."

The laughing stopped. The nurses were still. They bowed their heads over their lunches. And that's where we left it, knowing that denial is strongest in the women who have a need to protect themselves from having their secret exposed. While guarding their own secrets and defending their profession, many nurses unfortunately become enablers of hysterectomy.

After protesting alone on the third day, I drove into the country to see rural Mississippi. It was dark by the time I noticed the "low fuel" light. There were no cars for miles and miles on a lonely two-lane road with no streetlights, but then the headlights of a car appeared out of nowhere in my rearview mirror. It came up behind me quickly. I have a good instinct for danger, and I felt anxious that this car stayed behind me when most people would've passed. And just when I finally spotted a gas station, the tank ran dry. I coasted up as far as I could, but short of the pumps. I got out, put my shoulder to the frame, and started inching the car forward. The car following me stopped too, and without a word a large woman got out and put her shoulder to the passenger side, helping me push it the rest of the way.

"I'm sorry for following you, but I wanted to know about that sign," she said breathlessly.

As I filled up my tank, I told her about our protest in Jackson. "Well, it's too late for me," she said. "I suspected all along my problems weren't 'all in my head' like the doctor said."

I gave her one of the pamphlets, thanked her for her help, and told her to call HERS if she needed to speak with me. She sat in her car reading it. As she drove away she yelled, "God bless you for what you're doing."

The environment surrounding hysterectomy and the culture of how women live with it was different wherever we went. What remained universal was the damage it left in its wake. It was okay for a woman to risk an accident veering across an 8-lane street to get a brochure and a few words about hysterectomy through a car window. It was okay to run us off the road to get information or to follow me for miles and miles just to have a word with me. But it wasn't okay to be identified in public as a damaged woman.

It's a common fact of life for many hysterectomized women. They're open and honest with me over the phone when they call HERS. They often provide intimate details about their lives and relationships. I educate them about female anatomy and the functions of the female organs. But for a woman to hold a sign proclaiming that her sex organs were removed is another matter entirely. It's like having a scarlet H branded across your forehead. While some might think Mississippi women are naïve, the reason they don't talk about hysterectomy has nothing to do with naïvete—it's because they haven't been educated and informed about the functions of the female organs.

I could've spent an entire year in Jackson, doing nothing but giving information to women seeking validation that they weren't alone. I left Jackson feeling sick that we had to leave. But it was time to move on. Little did I know this would be the place that would need information more than any other city we'd visit.

FOUR

Nurses and doctors' wives.

Seattle, Washington—Rick Schweikert

When Nora told me that women sometimes send HERS photos of themselves before and after hysterectomy, I didn't think too much about it. Until, at the premiere of *un becoming* in New York, a woman with tears in her eyes thanked me, saying, "You're probably going to think I'm crazy, but can I show you a picture of me before the surgery?" And then after the next show it happened again. A woman who was married to a doctor said, "This is me before the surgery." We spoke with women all over the country who carry around photos to remind themselves of who they were before a doctor removed their female organs.

The biggest difference I notice in the photos is their eyes. As one woman explained, she showed me her photo to prove that before the surgery she was strong, vibrant, healthy, and happy, "When I still had that glint in my eyes."

The main protagonist in *un becoming* is an artist named Emma Douglas. She's a painter who refers to her work as her life's breath. She's married to an anesthesiologist named Sam Morgan. Sam's best friend happens to be Dr. James Ridge, the gynecologist who recommends "exploratory" surgery to Emma. Halley Ridge, Dr. Ridge's wife, was hysterectomized by her husband's colleague, but the audience doesn't discover that until the end of the play. In the end, Halley helps Emma avoid the surgery.

un becoming places accountability for hysterectomy on the shoulders of those who are most responsible. The villain of the

play is a gynecologist, and the hero is a hysterectomized woman—
his wife. This scenario had never been portrayed in any stage production before. When actors first picked up the script, they sometimes found the story hard to believe, as was the case with one of
the members of the Seattle cast. But it's unfortunately a common
story.

What follows is an excerpt from one of the thousands of
emails we've received from women whose lives mirror the story of
un becoming:

> Hi there,
> My name is… I am from… My doctor who
> I loved and never questioned, suggested a
> hysterectomy. He didn't think me being only
> 30 years old was an issue since I was married
> and had…children. He explained that I would
> take an estrogen pill each day, and basically I
> would be good as gold. (Not his words) that
> is how he made it seem. NO SIDE AFFECTS
> WERE EVER MENTIONED! I was told it would
> be no different than my c section surgeries as
> far as the pain was concerned. My mother had
> a hysterectomy…and told me that it would take
> a year before I felt better, however she had no
> idea what she would live the rest of her life like
> either. I…am having joint pain in my hands,
> knees, elbows and back. Before the hysterec-
> tomy I was fine, due to the pain I can no longer
> roller skate with my children, dance around the
> house and I fear that I am going to have to close
> my business. The list of side effects since the
> hysterectomy is too long…to put in this e-mail.
> This morning out of desperation…I found your
> site. I am beside myself thinking I am only go-
> ing to get worse. I am an artist and yesterday
> I couldn't hold the paint brush to paint at my
> easel, typing this e-mail is painful. What can I

do? Do you have any info that might help me?
Is there anyone else going through this?
Thank you for your time.
Sincerely,
(name and other identifiers omitted for confidentiality)

There have been a few books, such as Mary Daly's *GYN/ECOLOGY*, that accurately portray the life-altering effects of hysterectomy.[15] But most books on the subject ultimately twist the truth around to benefit the self-serving interests of its author, the publisher, or the university or pharmaceutical company that sponsored the author's research. *un becoming* is the story of hysterectomy told through the eyes of women—not the medical industrial establishment that targets them. The story is fictional, but two of the women who joined the protest in Seattle reminded us that the imaginary plot and characters are based on common experiences.

During the protests and talkbacks after the play, we met hundreds of hysterectomized women who were either nurses or the wives of doctors. And if that woman herself was an attorney or a nurse, audiences were shocked to hear that even that wasn't enough to protect them. Nora often says, "The greatest number of hysterectomy scars are worn by the wives of doctors. Second is nurses."

One of the women who joined us in Seattle was a writer who wrote a book about the before-and-after of hysterectomy. Her friend Fran (name changed for confidentiality) told her the story of how she ended up on an operating table. Fran was a registered nurse whose husband was a doctor. The surgeon who performed

[15] Daly, Mary, *GYN/ECOLOGY*, Beacon, 1990.

the "exploratory surgery" on her was the father of her daughter's close friend. All were in agreement that no organs were to be removed. She previously had one of her ovaries removed for an ordinary cyst, and she and her husband specifically made it clear that under no circumstances were the uterus or the remaining ovary to be removed. After the operation the surgeon emerged from the operating room, announcing that he had "excised the problem." Fran's husband, waiting for news about the surgery, was relieved…until the surgeon informed him that although he didn't remove her uterus he did remove her remaining ovary, against their expressed wishes.

As medical professionals, Fran and her husband knew that ovarian function is critical to health and wellbeing. Uterine function and viability depends on ovarian function. By removing Fran's remaining ovary, they knew that her hormone-responsive uterus would atrophy.

In order to keep her uterus viable, Fran was prescribed high levels of exogenous hormones—that is, hormones produced outside of her body. But while the endogenous hormones (produced naturally within her body) were beneficial to her, the exogenous hormones came with a host of dangers. The increased risk of cancer (breast, ovarian, uterine, and others), stroke, heart disease, dementia, and so on have been well-documented in studies and in literature.[16] Because of the adverse effects of high doses of hormones, coupled with the devastating physical loss of ovarian function (the predictable aftereffects of castration), Fran was now unable to control her emotions. So she was prescribed potent an-

---

[16] Women's Health Initiative, 1991-2006 study of 161,000 women; Seaman, Barbara, *The Greatest Experiment Ever Performed On Women*, Hyperion, 2004.

ti-depressants and other anxiety-controlling drugs with unknown potential interactions.

The betrayal of trust by her profession filled her with rage and despair. Nora says the angriest women who contact HERS are nurses and the wives of doctors. She was both. Her rage consumed her.

When she and her husband attended a HERS conference in Dallas a few years later, she said her medical records showed there was nothing of significance wrong with the first ovary the doctor had removed, and the remaining ovary was also healthy when he removed it.

In the end, the couple sued the doctor. It was a fairly blatant case of a high-handed doctor mutilating a woman against her expressed wishes. But she lost the lawsuit. The jury favored the doctor's word over hers and determined that the mutilating surgery had met the current "accepted standard of care." As the surgeon's defense attorney put it, her husband was a doctor and she was a nurse, so they should've known better.

Once the doctor became focused on Fran's benign ovarian cyst—a natural variation that required no treatment—a cascade of devastating decisions and actions ensued. Menstruating women produce an ovarian cyst every month. It's normal for the ovaries to develop physiologic (or functional) cysts when they ovulate midcycle, which wax and wane larger before menstruation and smaller after menstruation—usually a functional cyst develops on the right ovary one month, and on the left ovary the next month.

Other common, benign, ovarian cysts include dermoid, endometrioma (also called "chocolate" cysts), borderline, and teratoma. Dermoid cysts are rarely a cause for concern. They're primordial cysts that usually contain hair, teeth, and often fat. Like endometrioma, dermoid cysts tend to grow bilaterally (on both ovaries), but they can also develop on only one ovary. They can occur on the outside of the ovary on a stalk that extends from the ovary (its blood supply), or they can occur inside the ovary, encapsulated. Women are often told that the ovary with the cyst must be removed, but this begins with the faulty premise that the development of these cysts requires action. In fact, except for borderline cysts, which have a small incidence of becoming cancerous, these cysts are benign—they don't become malignant. Although they can become quite large, they may never cause a symptom. If they don't bother you, there's no reason to do anything about them. The worst-case scenario is they can rupture, but cysts don't rupture spontaneously—usually only through some kind of trauma to the abdomen, such as a forceful blow to the pelvis. If they do rupture, surgery is performed to irrigate the pelvis, which removes the contents of the cyst.

If the cyst is causing problems you can't live with, a cystectomy (surgical removal of the cyst) can usually be performed without removing the ovary—if the surgeon has the skill to do so. Ovaries are very resilient. They can be cut into pieces (called a wedge resection), the cyst removed, the pieces of the ovary sutured back together, and the ovary usually functions normally again.

If a cyst grows very large, some women feel pelvic pressure internally or they might experience urinary frequency. But usually they present no symptoms and are detected incidentally during a pelvic exam. Some women are especially prone to developing dermoid or endometrioma cysts, and after they're removed they may develop them over and over again. This is a time when they're especially vulnerable to hysterectomy, which is one reason to not go down the surgical path to begin with.

A Pap smear performed during a so-called well-woman visit is all too often an invitation to unnecessary treatment. The incidence of cancer in the female and the male sex organs is nearly identical, but men don't have their sex organs routinely inspected. And if doctors are hysterectomizing and castrating more than half a million healthy women each year, clearly the safe thing to do is to stay away from doctors and hospitals...even if you're a nurse and your husband is a doctor.

Hospitals are dangerous places. We're certainly not the first ones to say so. Nor was Robert S. Mendelsohn, an M.D. who was the President of the National Health Federation, the director of a hospital in Chicago, and a medical school professor:

> I have always told my patients that they should avoid hospitals as they would avoid a war. Do your utmost to stay out of them and, if you find yourself in one, do everything possible to get out as soon as you can. After working in hospitals for most of my life, I can assure you that they are the dirtiest and most deadly places in town.[17]

It would be ideal if we were all informed of these basic facts. But informing women about the irreversible aftermath of hysterectomy is bad for business, so we can't wait for doctors to do it. Women don't know better because doctors neglect to inform them. The vast majority of the women who call HERS cancel their

---

[17] Robert S. Mendelsohn, *MALePRACTICE*, Contemporary Books, 1981.

surgeries after they learn about female anatomy and the functions of the female organs.

"My doctor told me I was endangering my children by not having a hysterectomy," a woman told us during a talkback. "If I didn't have the surgery, he said, I was going to die and I wouldn't see my children grow up."

"So what did you do?" I asked.

"Nora knows," she said, "because she looked at my medical records with me, and there wasn't anything wrong with me."

"How long ago was that?"

"Fourteen years ago. My kids are in college, and I'm the picture of health."

If we heard it once we heard it a thousand times—"I canceled my surgery," women tell us, "and now I'm the picture of health. So why did my doctor tell me I needed a hysterectomy?"

The most frightening lines in *un becoming* found their way into the play because they're the things women tell us over and over again about what their doctors told them. They're repeated from coast-to-coast, from border-to-border, to women born a hundred years apart. While I was working on the first draft of *unbecoming*, my friend's mother yelled to him while he was on the phone with me, saying, "Tell Rick to put in his play what my doctor told me! Tell him my doctor said, 'Don't worry, I'm just taking out the crib, but I'm leaving the playpen.'"

In other words, women aren't able to bear children after hysterectomy, but their sexual partners will still have a vaginal pocket for intercourse, even though a loss of sexual feeling is an anatomical fact for hysterectomized women. So I did put it into the play…but only after I heard that same line a dozen or more times. We continue to hear it from women all over the country, including right there in the state of Washington. These one-liners from gynecologists trivialize women's concerns about their sex organs as they sit half-naked on examination tables.

Women are told to eat nothing after midnight the night before the surgery and to get their things in order because they'll be out of commission for a while as they "recover." But recovery presumes they'll be the same person after the surgery as they were before, which isn't possible. What they're not told is far more important than what they are told. It's what isn't being said that's really at issue here.

One of the protestors who joined us in Seattle was an attorney. Her expertise was drafting language that could be defended in court. She was diagnosed with uterine cancer and consented to a hysterectomy, but not castration. It might seem foolish for a doctor to castrate a bright attorney, who not only modified the hospital's consent form to reflect her wishes prior to the hysterectomy but also included specific language expressly stating that under no circumstances were her ovaries to be removed. And yet, like the nurse mentioned above, against her wishes a doctor removed her ovaries anyway.

She wanted to sue, but no attorney would take the case because most states have a "reasonable person" or "a reasonable physician" standard. The lawyers advised her that the courts would assume that once she entered the hospital, any *reasonable* physician would've chosen to castrate her while hysterectomizing her—even if it was contrary to her written wishes. If you enter a hospital in a reasonable-physician statute state, your wishes may mean nothing.

The courts will very likely support whatever the doctor deems is reasonable.

The issue boils down to whether a woman has the right to decide what will be done to her body. The Constitution of the United States guarantees personal sovereignty, and our government exists to protect it. When informed consent is missing from the decision making process, personal sovereignty is denied to women. Decisions about what women will and won't allow to be done to their bodies should never be taken away from them, under any circumstances.

On the first day of the Seattle protest we turned our signs toward the Swedish Medical Center instead of the traffic, so the doctors and patients inside the building could see them. Massive cranes loomed overhead, a sign that business was booming.

That evening a reading of *un becoming* was hosted by the Women's Studies Department at the University of Washington in a lecture hall on campus. Like the cast, a few people in the talkback had a difficult time accepting that doctors knowingly harm women. It's an unattractive side of human nature that most people are unwilling to attribute to doctors.

"So who's to blame?" I asked them. As with most audiences, someone said, "I think women need to educate themselves." But what does that have to do with whether or not doctors knowingly harm women? And who could possibly be more educated on these issues than a nurse and a doctor? A medical education didn't save her. Isn't that what we pay doctors for, to advise us on issues we don't have time to go to medical school to learn?

Although it's rare for a doctor to be prosecuted in a criminal court for harming patients, the *Seattle Times* reported the case of a King County gynecologist convicted of two counts of rape and two counts of "indecent liberties" against four Seattle women who testified against him. The last lines of the *Times* article read, "Momah remains charged with three counts of health-care fraud, which will be tried later. In addition, he faces civil suits from dozens of women who say he sexually abused them or botched surgeries." Such cases are common, and for every one we do hear about, how many more are there that we don't hear about?[18]

Insurance fraud is a criminal offense that is punishable by imprisonment. The unconsented removal of women's sex organs, though, is a civil offense that usually goes unpunished even in the most blatant cases. To find out why, follow the money. What's a uterus worth? Not much. But what's hysterectomy—the 20-30 minute surgery to remove the uterus—worth to hospitals and doctors? Tens of billions of dollars each year. And what are the male sex organs worth? It's worth searching for a man's penis in the dirt and spending nine hours in the operating room reattaching it, as was the case when Lorena Bobbit severed John Wayne Bobbit's penis after he raped her in 1993.[19]

Another woman who attended the protest and the play with her husband said they were both grateful to HERS for helping her remain intact. A doctor tried to badger her into letting him hysterectomize her. She sought other opinions, but one doctor after another supported the first doctor's recommendation, until she found HERS.

Nora was interviewed by a local television station in Seattle, but the hospital administrators at Swedish were smarter than some

---

[18] Ostrom, Carol M., "Momah Found Guilty of Sexual Crimes Against Patients," *Seattle Times*, November 16, 2005.
[19] "Bobbitt arrested on domestic violence charge," *CNN.com*, May 14, 2002.

hospitals we'd been to. They didn't call the police, so we didn't have flashing lights to draw attention to our protest.

We spoke with a woman who said she was afraid because she couldn't keep up with the minimum payments she was required to make to Swedish to pay down the debt incurred when she was hysterectomized there without health insurance. Meanwhile, the Swedish website says not only can you make a donation to Swedish, "If you would prefer to pledge a fixed amount on a regular basis, call us and we can help you set up an automatic contribution plan."

It's an ugly game of round robin. Surgeons' wives are hysterectomized, as well as the nurses who assist them in surgery. Indigent women are put on payment plans to pay for unnecessary hysterectomies, or taxpayers are sent the bill via Medicaid and Medicare. The public is encouraged to set up automatic contribution plans to pad the medical industry's bottom line and help pay surgeons exorbitant payoffs for doing this grisly work. And then the courts protect the doctors and hospital administrators when suits are brought against them, because unwarranted surgery has become the standard of care. Health and wellbeing has almost nothing to do with it.

FIVE

The history of hysterectomy and female castration.

Little Rock, Arkansas—Nora W. Coffey

Hello Nora,

I just received your news letter regarding the
next event. I am so sad that I can not attend any
of them. I would love to however, I am disabled
due to "UNNECESSARY AND UNAUTHOR-
IZED" hysterectomy that was done on me in
1976 at the age of 25. I have had problems ever
since this was done to me and I am 100% behind
your movement, even though I may not benefit
from it. Maybe others can be protected. I am living on a very low fixed income and am unable
to travel anywhere due to lack of funds but my
thoughts and prayers are with you all. I admire
you for doing what you are doing. Unfortunately,
the butcher that did my surgery is dead now
so there is nothing I can do about the violent
crime committed against me. I am only 52 years
old and my life is ruined. Has been for quite
some time and all because of that surgery. I was
told I was going to have a laparoscopy ONLY,
that was "ALL" that I signed for, when I awoke
they had removed both ovaries, both tubes, my
uterus and my appendix !!!!! I was extremely
confused, frightened and devastated !!!
Anyway, I just wanted to thank you for all your
hard work for this very important and just cause
and say my thoughts and prayers are will all of
you working on this issue. GOD bless you all,
–(name omitted for confidentiality)

Lois and I agreed to meet near the University of Arkansas
for Medical Sciences Medical Center—"one of the largest public

employers in the state" [20]—practically a self-regulating city unto itself.

The location turned out to be not so good of a location for a protest, and we were there for only a short while before the police showed up. The officer seemed interested in what we were doing, though, and wasn't in the least bit confrontational, even suggesting an alternate location on an eight-lane road in view of anyone driving into or out of the hospital.

Little Rock was the first city where we played red light/green light to get our information into the hands of the public. When the cars lined up at the red light, we passed by each one offering them a pamphlet. When the light turned green we returned to the sidewalk to give pamphlets to anyone who might be walking by. There were more cars than I could possibly reach before the light changed, but it didn't take long for Lois to catch on to it too, and soon we were handing out a lot of information.

Most people we offered information to took it. They were pleasant, but not particularly chatty. They took our pamphlets with blank expressions on their faces, then put their windows back up and drove away. During one of the green lights, Lois mentioned that her daughter drove by. It seemed a little odd she didn't stop to greet us.

I had counseled Lois on the phone, but it was clearly a relief for her to talk with someone in person. She lived in a small town quite a distance from Little Rock. "No one in my town even says the word 'hysterectomy'," she said. But that didn't keep her from talking about the impact the surgery had on her and her family.

[20] http://www.uams.edu/chancellor/about.asp.

She knew of a lot of women who denied that the surgery had changed their lives, but Lois knew that couldn't be true. Although there was no one for her to speak with, she never doubted that other women felt the same way she did. Even still, the first time that was confirmed was when she contacted HERS.

Most women who have no one to validate their experiences begin to doubt themselves. Lois understood that the women who denied their experiences did so because they didn't want others to know they were struggling. It's a well-guarded secret—feeling exhausted, in pain, with a loss of sexual feeling and vitality that makes every day a struggle aren't characteristics that make most women feel good about themselves. Most of us want to feel sensual, energetic, healthy, and strong. If Lois' neighbors were able to talk openly about their loss of sexuality and sexual feeling, what would happen to their intimate relationships? If they told people they were struggling from profound pain and fatigue, who'd hire them?

When you visit rural communities where few women feel they can afford such honest discussions, it's easy to see why hysterectomy is one of history's best-kept secrets.

The story of how hysterectomy has become the standard of care for a host of benign conditions goes back many centuries. Some feminist scholars, like Mary Daly, begin with the patriarchal creation myths, what Daly calls "The Sado-Ritual Syndrome: The Re-Enactment of Goddess Murder."[21] Other medical historians begin with the surgical experimentations of J. Marion Sims, or by going back further to Hippocrates.

---

[21] Daly, Mary, *GYN/ECOLOGY*, Beacon, 1990.

Hippocrates is the ancient Greek physician who is often referred to as "the father of modern medicine," credited with what is now called the Hippocratic Oath. Hippocrates helped set the tone for more than 2,000 years of gynecology when he asked, "What is woman?" He then answered his own question: "Disease."

Some ancient physicians believed that the womb was actually a sort of beast, capable of wandering around inside of women. This theory gave rise to the "wandering womb" myth. Hippocrates himself believed that hysteria was caused by a wandering uterus. And if the womb of an ancient Greek woman was believed to have risen up out of her pelvis, a physician might try to make it go back down to where it was supposed to be by tying a putrid-smelling substance to the woman's face and putting flowers on her vagina. As crazy as it may sound to us today, in this way, they thought, the uterus would recoil away from the putrid smell toward the flowery smell and that would end the hysteria.

It's no wonder that five hundred years before the birth of Christ and a hundred years before Hippocrates was born, Heraclitus of Ephesus said, "Doctors cut, burn, and torture the sick, and then demand of them an undeserved fee for such services." Apparently, being sick itself wasn't a prerequisite for "medical" experimentation.

The first known hysterectomy experiment was performed by Soranus of Ephesus in the 2nd century AD.[22] The woman died during the procedure. Other surgeons attempted to surgically remove the uterus, but most of the rest of the millennia would go by before a woman would actually survive one.

[22] Vietz, P. F., "Hysterectomy—A Historical Perspective," http://www.qis.net/~pvietz/history.htm, September 1997.

The first known reference to the correlation between the uterus and female sexuality came from a Renaissance-era Italian physician. Although no woman had yet survived the surgery, Jacopo Berengario DaCarpi correctly surmised that a loss of sexual feeling was an inevitable aftereffect of hysterectomy. Because of a long history of male castration, the consequences of removing the male sex organs had been well-documented. So it made sense to expect the same from removing the female organs. And yet up to the present day most doctors continue to deny any association between the uterus and sexuality, although DaCarpi got it right 500 years ago when he guessed that women, like their male counterparts, would lose their sexual vigor when their sex organs were removed.[23]

The medical record is spotty, but medical historians have investigated the tragic history of hysterectomy. Guy I. Benrubi credits C. J. M. Langenbeck in Gottingen, Germany with the first "modern hysterectomy" in 1813. According to Benrubi:

> It is also probably the first case of total vaginal hysterectomy where the patient survived... Despite Langenbeck's success this operation was so fraught with morbidity and mortality that for many years it was not an accepted procedure... [In his second hysterectomy] a sponge was again left in the vagina, and 20 leaches were applied on the abdomen to relieve abdominal pain. The patient died on the second postoperative day.[24]

The first American hysterectomy was performed by John Collins Warren of Boston in 1829. The patient died four days later.

---

[23] Berengario da Carpi, Jacopo, *Isagogae Breves*, Benedetto Faelli, 1523.
[24] Benrubi, Guy I., "History of Hysterectomy," *Journal of the Florida Medical Association*, August 1988.

Benrubi reports that the procedure fell out of favor from 1830 to 1850, because the technique "often led to rectal and bladder injuries and the cause of death was peritonitis."

Bear in mind, the first widely recognized use of anesthesia was Crawford Long's use of ether in 1842.[25] Most of the women who "survived" most likely died from complications, if not from the illness the surgery was intended to treat. Hysterectomy should've been abandoned right then and there. According to Benrubi, some doctors attempted to convince their colleagues to do just that:

> An example of the discontent with which this operation was met is exemplified by the writing of Dieffenback, one of the greatest German surgeons of his time (1792-1847): 'To take the entire womb from the belly of a woman means the removal of that woman's soul… Still, some daring men attempt it and they deserve our thanks in as much as the results of their terrible operation furnish us all the proof needed to banish this procedure from the field of surgery. According to my opinion, an indication for this operation does not exist. The attempted extirpation of the womb partakes more of the character of murder tales than of curative surgical operations.'

Feminist scholar Mary Daly notes two horrific moments in 19th century gynecological history. The first is the "invention" of clitoridectomy (removal of the clitoris) by British gynecologist Isaac Baker Brown. Brown's genital mutilation procedure was "enthusiastically accepted as a 'cure' for female masturbation," Daly writes. The second development came in 1873, with Robert Battey's use of oophorectomy (removal of the ovaries, female castration) "to

---

[25] Boland, Frank Kels, *The First Anesthetic: The Story of Crawford Long*, University of Georgia Press, 1950.

cure insanity and to 'elevate the moral sense of the patients, making them tractable, orderly, industrious, and cleanly.'"[26]

Walter Burnham performed over 300 oophorectomies from 1851 to 1882. Burnham performed the first "successful" female castration, but about one of every four of his patients died. To paraphrase a quote by playwright George Bernard Shaw, a gynecologist's reputation was made by the number of women who died under his care.

In 1880, the mortality rate for hysterectomy was estimated at a staggering 70 percent. Despite these figures, by 1914, the Mayo Clinic recommended vaginal hysterectomy for the repair of cystocele, which is a prolapsed or sagging bladder. It's a benign condition for which hysterectomy never needs to be performed unless you have the wrong doctor and the wrong hospital. And yet it's clear that modern medicine had by the 20th century embraced hysterectomy as the "common" surgical procedure it is today.

Hysterectomy experimentation isn't just a thing of the past. It continues today with the use of robots to remove the uterus. Women remain the ultimate test animal, and it's telling that Benrubi's account of the history of "the profession" concludes with gynecology's ongoing search for an alibi to "redefine the indications" for hysterectomy. [27]

There are other gynecological pioneers who should be mentioned, such as J. Marion Sims, who has been called the "father of gynecology" or the "architect of the vagina." Daly says this of Sims:

> He was an object of adulation at Harvard Medical School, where "the students recognized 'divinity' in Sims and counted him 'one

---

[26] Daly, ibid.
[27] Benrubi, ibid.

of the immortals.'" As Peggy Holland has remarked, such men are "immortals" in the sense
that they pass on death and fear, their only true
offspring.[28]

John Archer tells us in *Bad Medicine*[29] that Sims purchased
slaves for his experimental surgeries. One of these women endured
30 surgeries without any anesthesia before dying. In *Te Linde's
Operative Gynecology*, the section titled "Historical Development of
Pelvic Surgery" begins with a quote from Howard A. Kelly: "No
group should ever neglect to honor the work of forbears upon
which their contributions are based." Kelly says of Sims' work:

- "The term *experiments* is appropriate, since four years of
  experimentation elapsed before his first success."
- "He had no experience in pelvic surgery; in fact, he dis-
  liked it."
- "His many failures only stimulated his determination
  and efforts."
- "All his operations were done without asepsis and without anesthesia."
- "...Sims made one of the important surgical contributions of the 19th century..."

I found almost no mention anywhere in the history of hysterectomy about the women these men experimented on. There's
no effort at all by the authors of *Te Linde's* to memorialize the
unimaginable torture and suffering women endured.

There's a monument dedicated to Sims near the state
Capitol building in Columbia, South Carolina. The Medical University of South Carolina established the "J. Marion Sims Chair in

---

[28] Daly, ibid.
[29] Archer, John, *Bad Medicine*, Simon & Shuster, 1995.

Obstetrics-Gynecology." A dormitory at the University of South Carolina also bears his name. And Lancaster County's first regional hospital was named the Marion Sims Memorial Hospital. All of this for a man who wrote the following in his autobiography, *The Story of My Life*:

> I knew nothing about medicine, but I had sense enough to see that doctors were killing their patients; that medicine was not an exact science; that it was wholly empirical, and that it would be better to trust entirely to Nature than to the hazardous skills of the doctors.[30]

So he became one.

No history of gynecology would be complete without mentioning the Nazi doctors in WWII concentration camps. Nazi doctors like Joseph Mengele (known as "the Angel of Death" in Auschwitz), Dr. Horst Schumann (conducted untold numbers of sterilization/hysterectomy experiments at Auschwitz before his subjects succumbed to death), Dr. Carl Clauberg (sterilization/hysterectomy and castration experiments, s`Auschwitz), Dr. Viktor Brack (sterilization/hysterectomy experiments, Auschwitz), Dr. Dering (sterilization/hysterectomy experiments, Auschwitz), Dr. Hermann Stieve (studied menstrual cycles following torture, Plotensee Prison and Ravensbruck Concentration Camp), Dr. Adolph Porkorny (sterilization/hysterectomy experiments, Auschwitz), Dr. Siegfried Handloser (supervised all "treatments" conducted at Buchenwald), and Edward Wirths (the chief SS doctor), to name a few.[31]

Helmut and Edward Wirths implanted cancerous cells into the female organs of Jewish women in Nazi death camps and then

---

[30] Sims, J. Marion, *The Story of My Life*, D. Appleton & Company, 1884.
[31] Multiple sources, including Spitz, Vivien, *Doctor From Hell: The Horrific Account of Nazi Experiments on Humans*, Sentient Publications, 2005.

hysterectomized them so they could observe how the cancerous cells grew. Several accounts from holocaust survivors (and the diaries of those who didn't survive) recount these men having a charming and pleasant demeanor throughout their experiments, offering their terrified subjects a reassuring smile and a pleasant "there, there now." If a day ever comes when American doctors injure women in the name of medicine, you might say, then we'll know we're in serious trouble. But that day is here. The Food and Drug Administration, the American Medical Association, and the American College of Obstetricians and Gynecologists (ACOG) are all run by doctors. Gynecologists are all but immune from criminal or civil recourse. There's no governing body for gynecologists that doesn't have an inherent conflict of interest. How many more generations will it take for America to wake up to what's being done to women right here in our own hometowns?

In 1971, ACOG members met to discuss hysterectomy. More than 2,000 years after Hippocrates' death, gynecologist Ralph W. White said of the uterus, "It's a useless, bleeding, symptom-producing, potential cancer-bearing organ."[32] He was applauded by his fellow doctors. This statement is like an echo across the millennia from Hippocrates, who equated women with disease.

Given this long history of physicians' disregard for the health of women, it seems entirely appropriate for women like Lois to be angry toward the medical community. After our first day of protest in Little Rock, she asked to keep her protest sign she was carrying. When she got home she put it in her front yard.

Earlier that morning, Lois and her daughter picked me up at the hotel. Her daughter said little on the car ride over to

---

[32] Robbins, John, *Reclaiming Our Health*, H.J. Kramer, 1996.

the hospital. She offered only a brief hello when Lois introduced us. It turns out she was a nursing student there at the university's medical school. This wouldn't be the only time when the child of a protestor would be affiliated in some way with a medical center, a situation that was difficult for both of them. I did my best to inform prospective protestors, friends, and family that if any of them worked at the hospital we chose (or had a relative who worked there) we'd do our best to choose a different one, if that was a concern for them. As it turned out, this was only an issue twice—in Detroit and Los Angeles. Most of the protestors were pleased we'd be protesting in front of their local hospital.

The wind that first day made holding up our signs tricky. So when her daughter came to pick us up after the protest, Lois asked her to drive to an arts-and-crafts store to get some materials to tie the signs down to the street poles.

On the car ride to the store, I sat in the back of their SUV with the windows rolled down. Lois' daughter tried to be conversational with her mother, but I could sense a definite tension between them. Lois asked to stop at another store, leaving us in the car to talk. I asked if it made her uncomfortable to have us protesting at the medical center where she was a student. At first she was tentative and vague, but before long she began to share with me what it was like for her since her mother's surgery. How things had changed at home. The hurt was palpable, and under the hurt was anger. They clearly wanted and needed to talk and to hear each other's perspectives, but they couldn't.

And yet, in that brief conversation, I could feel that familiar shift that lets me know something's changing with a child's perception of her mom. She lowered her guard just a little when she realized I understood. I let her know it wasn't her fault, that she wasn't to blame for her response to the loss of the mother she knew before the surgery.

The next day, Lois and I were back in front of the hospital. Her daughter drove by, but this time she waved and motioned that she was parking the car. In a few minutes she was walking down the hill to join us. Lois didn't say a word, but she was obviously pleased.

As we handed out information through car windows, I could feel her daughter's eyes on me and something continuing to shift inside her. And then, after a few more minutes, she took a stack of pamphlets from the box. It wasn't long before she was running up to cars and giving out as much information as Lois and me combined.

The hurt and anger her daughter felt began to recede. A lot of that anger was most likely the result of confusion—an inability to understand her mother's pain and who was responsible for it.

There's no appropriate person for children of hysterectomized women to direct their anger at. Should they be angry with their mother for allowing herself to be hysterectomized? No, of course not. Her father? The doctor? Sure, a doctor did this to her mother, but like so many people she was socialized to respect doctors and not question their actions.

The Little Rock protest empowered Lois' daughter to question the people who make unconsented hysterectomy possible. It gave them a voice and a proactive environment to communicate about their shared loss.

SIX

"Is this where they hurt my momma?"

Baton Rouge, Louisiana—Nora W. Coffey

In Little Rock and Seattle we were joined by adult children of local protestors. In Baton Rouge I was joined by Judy and her three young children, which was an altogether different experience. In a way that only a child can view it—without the distraction of feeling compelled to reduce it to an intellectual concern—these children were vocal and inquisitive about hysterectomy.

Having met in the parking lot, I walked with the oldest child, Judy's son, to our protest site at the Baton Rouge Woman's Hospital. I carried one of the "Hysterectomy Damages Women" signs, and along the way, he asked, "Miss, what does that word mean?"

I gave him a brief definition of *hysterectomy*.

"And that word…what does that mean?" he asked, pointing to another word on the sign.

I explained what *damages* means.

Then the boy turned to Judy and asked her to define the words on her sign. Finally, he asked me, "Is this the hospital where they hurt my momma?"

"Yes," Judy said, "this is the place where the doctor hurt your momma."

His age is about the right age to begin educating children about anatomy—just as soon as they're mature enough to comprehend the language. Judy's children understood the need to ask questions before accepting help from strangers.

Most of us seek medical help with the expectation of a uniform standard of care. Unfortunately that's a dangerous presumption to make. That's why it's so important to learn how to choose a doctor.

If you have symptoms, to determine if any treatment should be considered it's important to know what studies and tests should be utilized to evaluate them. The first step is to decide if you should see a gynecologist who specializes in looking for irregularities in the female organs, or if you should see a whole body doctor, since your female organs are part of your whole-body system. Gynecology is a surgical sub-specialty, so it makes sense that they're predisposed to surgery.

Most doctors' reputations are based on personality and marketing, and not expertise. So the best way to find a doctor is by asking people you know who are healthy and who haven't undergone unwarranted surgery or invasive treatments. Asking for a referral from people who have undergone surgery might result in finding a doctor who is predisposed to invasive treatments.

To choose a doctor with good outcomes it helps to learn what questions to ask and the correct answers to those questions. When choosing a doctor, knowing the right questions to ask won't help much, unless you know the answers. Only then can you evaluate the doctor's response. Children are taught to be wary of anyone who is reluctant to answer their questions, and so should adults.

For example, a woman might ask a gynecologist, "Is removal of the ovaries castration?" The correct answer is yes, the medically correct term for removal of the gonads is castration. Or a woman might ask, "Are hysterectomized women at a greater risk of heart disease?" Again, the correct answer is yes, it's well documented that hysterectomized women have a three times greater incidence of myocardial infarction and a seven times greater risk if the ovaries are also removed.[33] Knowing the answers to these questions equips women with valuable information to appraise the prospective doctor's honesty, integrity, and knowledge of the facts.

In the Colorado chapter of this book, you'll find a discussion about what questions to ask a prospective doctor when considering a myomectomy for the removal of fibroids. Asking a doctor if he or she is aware of the HERS Foundation might be informative. Observing the doctor's response while reviewing the information provided on the HERS website or bringing this book with you to your next consultation might also prove quite helpful.

Judy's kids standing there with us in front of Baton Rouge Woman's Hospital must've been quite a sight. We got some curious looks from people driving by. The youngest one draped her teddy bear over her sign. More than in any other city, people in Baton Rouge stopped to ask us, "What's this all about?"

It was an insufferably hot and humid day in southern Louisiana. The midday sun was scorching. The children were hot and tired. Before long they wandered over to a park bench in the shade. The youngest asked me for a pencil and began writing on one of the pamphlets. After a while, one of the girls jumped down from the park bench and approached me.

The pamphlets we handed out had four true/false questions printed on the front cover:

---

[33] Centerwall, Brandon S., "Premenopausal hysterectomy and cardiovascular disease," *American Journal of Obstetrics and Gynecology*, January 1, 1981; Rosenberg, Lynn et al, "Early menopause and the risk of myocardial infarction," *American Journal of Obstetrics and Gynecology*, 1981.

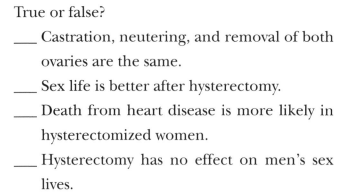

True or false?

___ Castration, neutering, and removal of both ovaries are the same.

___ Sex life is better after hysterectomy.

___ Death from heart disease is more likely in hysterectomized women.

___ Hysterectomy has no effect on men's sex lives.

The youngest child handed me the pamphlet she was writing on. All around the borders she'd drawn hearts and "to nora," inverting some of the letters—one of the many precious souvenirs of the Protest & Play year. "My sister read me all the questions," she said. "Did I get them right?"

They were too young to understand what "sex life" meant, but they understood that nothing is better after hysterectomy. They also understood that heart disease is bad and that hysterectomy was bad for their mother. So if it hurt their mother, then it hurt them, so it must be bad for everyone. And indeed, this little girl with her teddy bear in tow answered every question correctly. I thought about the doctors I've been interviewed with on major television talk shows who don't answer those questions accurately. Quite proud of herself, she returned to the bench in the shade.

In 1982 when I founded HERS, the word "hysterectomized" didn't exist. HERS coined it because, after all, women don't do it to themselves. The word "hysterectomy" itself was rarely spoken in public then. It was in the closet, in the dark, and no organization existed to encourage women to talk truthfully and openly about what had been done to them and the suffering they endured at the hands of doctors.

One misconception is that women with little formal education and poor women are more likely to undergo unnecessary hysterectomy than more educated and wealthy women. We met women on the Protest & Play tour who were wealthy and educated at the highest levels who took extraordinary measures to protect themselves from doctors…to no avail.

Every woman is unique and every woman's way of understanding information is unique. HERS approach to providing information is comprehensive. We break down the common barriers to learning. We're committed to figuring out how each woman best receives information and to provide information in such a way that each woman can understand and utilize it.

HERS empowers women with the information necessary to make decisions about what they will and won't consent to be done to their bodies. HERS demystifies information, translates emails from foreign languages, conferences-in translators for counseling calls, and reduces unfamiliar medical jargon into plain English. HERS acts as a liaison between women and doctors. We remind women their age isn't a disease. We help women differentiate medical problems from nuisances. We inform them about the alternatives and risks of treatment options, and we help women understand their anatomy and what happens when the female organs are removed. That is full disclosure.

HERS is an effective working model that demonstrates that it's possible for every woman to fully understand even the most complex information about her anatomy and why the female organs are vital to her health and well-being her entire lifetime, irrespective of her age, desire for children, or socio-economic status.

HERS debunks the commonly stated position that too much information is confusing and that women only need a limited amount of information. The surgery can't be undone—the damage is permanent. There's no such thing as too much information. Women must be fully informed before they're told to sign a Hysterectomy Consent form, or it's not *informed* consent.

Some people have said the HERS website and educational materials make them angry or frightened. These are appropriate responses. We all should be angry about what gynecologists are doing to women. Pain, sexual loss, and isolation are the daily reality of most of the more than 22 million hysterectomized women alive today. And there are things we should all be afraid of. Fear is a natural mechanism that alerts us to danger.

We all need to listen to the voice of intuition in such moments, but we also need full disclosure of accurate information.

Being a mother myself who was hysterectomized and castrated when my children were quite young, I thought about what this protest might mean to Judy and her kids. The hospital must've loomed gigantic before them. Two security guards—a man and a woman, slightly menacing, slightly silly looking—emerged from the hospital to tell us to leave.

Judy's children seemed unperturbed by the security guards. From the looks on their faces, they knew the security guards were wrong. They knew this was the right place to be. Being out there empowered them, like they were standing up for their mother and the mothers of other children. But they were also torn. They were well-behaved children who were raised to respect elders and authority. Their dilemma over how to react to the security guards was like so many of us in the doctor's office, not wanting to make the doctor angry by questioning their authority.

We often wonder if doctors will think we're questioning their judgment if we ask basic questions. Will they think we don't trust them if we ask them to talk with us about the options they don't offer?

Just like my own children at that age, the surgery cost Judy's children some of their innocence. They too would grow up questioning everything once they fully understood what a doctor had done to their mother.

When the security guards realized we had no intention of leaving, they barked at the children, saying they were sitting too close to the hospital. Judy's son knitted his eyebrows tighter as the security guards glared at us. He set his jaw again.

Judy and I explained that we wanted the children back there where they were safely away from the fast-moving traffic. The female guard repeated herself that the children wouldn't be allowed to sit so close to the hospital.

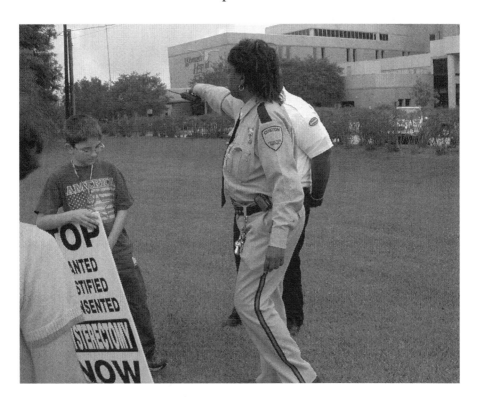

"So you want us to move the children closer to the traffic," I asked, "and put them into harm's way?"

"No," the security officer said, "you can just leave!"

"We're not leaving."

"Then keep the children off our property!" the officer said. And with that they made an about-face and returned to the air-conditioned halls of the hospital.

A little while later the female guard returned. She again told the children to stand in the sun near the traffic. But when the guard returned inside, the children wandered back to the bench, knowing neither Judy nor I would stop them.

Through it all Judy continued protesting. She said she hoped the doctor who operated on her would come out of the hospital. She wanted him to see what he'd done to her and how he'd hurt them as a family.

Several protestors went inside the hospitals we protested at to look for the doctor who had removed their sex organs. Many of them would protest for that reason—an opportunity to confront the doctor while surrounded by the support of other protestors. They wanted to say, "This is what you did to me. What kind of a person would do this to a woman?"

But no, none of the cowards in Baton Rouge or any other city would come out to speak with us. They were inside hiding behind the protection of the law. All over the country, doctors and nurses from hospital departments outside of gynecology would speak with us, but almost never a gynecologist, except to make some mean or spiteful remark while quickly hurrying by us. Why? Because they couldn't defend what they were doing to women.

The protest was a catalyst for families to talk about how the surgery impacted their lives. Questions they didn't have the vocabulary to ask became the key to unlocking doors of understanding. Like a locked room at the end of the hall, once a woman and her family understood how to open the door, anger and silence were slowly replaced with understanding. Life would never be anything like what it was before the surgery, but it was always a great relief for the door of communication to finally be opened.

It was scary at first for the protesters, mostly because they couldn't go back in time and "unknow" what they learned about hysterectomy. But the mothers invariably seemed closer with their children after finding the language to talk about the H word. You could see the anger melt away as they began to understand.

Earlier in the day, Judy's son accompanied me to the store to get a cold drink. "I'm really mad," he said suddenly.

"Why?" I asked.

"Because they really hurt my momma."

SEVEN

Follow the money.

St. Louis, Missouri—Rick Schweikert

When we arrived in St. Louis the skies were clear. The weather changed quickly though, and a cold, driving rain caught us off guard.

We didn't see any other protestors waiting to brave the torrential storm, so we stayed in the car rather than set up the protest in a deluge. But then right on time Joy showed up prepared for come what may.

Joy was a postal worker, and she joked that neither rain nor heat nor snow nor gloom of night would stop HERS from educating the public. Even in a driving rainstorm, Joy was a pleasure to protest with.

Hundreds of cars pulled across two, three, or even four lanes to get information and thank us for what we were doing. One of the cars that pulled up was a BMW. But instead of another appreciative St. Louisan, the driver was a doctor with *Obstetrics & Gynecology* sewn onto the pocket of her white coat. She barked at me, referring to the pamphlet I was handing her, "I know what's in there! And you're stupid!"

I burst into laughter, but she just sat there glaring at me, so I dropped the pamphlet into her open window. It looked strange there on her rain-speckled, black leather seat.

I imagined the doctor's anger turned toward the women she'd see in her office that day. We knew the protests were difficult for some women, because it exposed how damaged they were by the surgery. But the protests were also difficult for doctors. By making the public aware, we were also putting the scarlet H onto the lab coats of the gynecologists of Barnes-Jewish Hospital.

The deluge was followed by a spectacular calm-after-the-storm, azure morning. I sat in the sunshine with my journal and a cup of coffee at a cafe in the Soulard District. The café was just around the corner from the Soulard Theatre Collective in a former Czechoslavakian social hall, where Hydeware Theatre would present a Sunday matinee reading of *un becoming.*

There were only five or six people in the audience, but who could blame anyone for choosing to be outside on such a glorious day? Even with that small audience, though, the play made an impact.

During the performance I watched the reactions of a woman who sat with a man just a few seats from me. She cringed, covered her mouth with her hand, slouched down in her chair, laughed, and then in the end sat up straight with her eyes wide. She clapped vigorously for the performance, and when Nora and I took the stage to take questions, she asked, "Where are the doctors?"

One of the cast members named Betsy had invited a female gynecologist who said she'd be there, but she didn't show. Betsy then asked Nora exactly what doctors do during the surgery.

When Nora talks about how a hysterectomy is performed, she speaks in plain layperson's English. But to me nothing's more telling than the actual medical descriptions used to describe the procedure. My explanatory notes are in brackets:

> A left paramedian incision was made with a sharp knife and carried through the subcutaneous tissue. [*"Para" in this usage means "along" and median is "middle," so the scalpel was pushed into her skin in the middle of the abdomen, starting probably just above the pubis and running up to the belly but-*

ton.] A few bleeders were clamped at this point and with a second knife the incision was carried through to the fascia [*a layer of tissue covering the muscles*] and extended in a superior inferior fashion. Bleeders were clamped and tied with #2-0 plain tie at that point. The fascia was identified and nicked around the muscle bed and then incised with a scissors in a superior and inferior fashion using forceps to pick it up and then the muscle was sharply and bluntly dissected off the medial edge of the fascia at the midline. The muscle was then separated bluntly in a superior and inferior fashion until the peritoneum [*the smooth membrane that lines the abdomen*] was identified. A few small bleeders were tied with stick-ties. The peritoneum was grasped with forceps and the peritoneum was then entered sharply and the incision was extended with Metzenbaum scissors in a superior and inferior fashion... The uterus was then grasped with Kelly clamps at the cornu on the left and the right and the free space was identified and the left and right round ligaments were tied with single stick ties and the bladder flap was created after excision of the round ligaments. [*He cut through the ligaments that held her uterus. One of them is the uterosacral ligament, which attaches to the uterus and the sacrum in the lower back and accounts for part of the reason why hysterectomized women have back problems.*] The bladder flap was brought down in the usual fashion, following which the clear space was identified on the left and entered bluntly. Kelly clamps were then placed across the infundibulopelvic ligament at this point... [*The infundibulopelvic ligament is the ovarian ligament. It's difficult to tell exactly when it took place, but somewhere in here he also cuts through the hypogastric plexus of nerves, which Te Linde's gynecology textbook tells us provides feeling*

to the clitoris (see page 22): "*This latter extension
contains the fibers that innervate the vestibular bulbs
and clitoris.*"] This area was then incised with
scissors, both on the right and on the left and
the pedicles were tied with #3-0 chromic free
tie and a single chromic stick tie. [*He cut around
the uterus.*] Following this Heaney clamps were
placed across the cervical isthmus [*Now only the
cardinal ligaments around the cervix hold the uterus
in place. He then clamps onto the cervix, which is the
opening or neck of the uterus that is continuous with
the vagina.*] at the level of the uterine arteries on
the left and the right and pedicles were **treated
with sharp knife** [*my emphasis*] and the pedicles
were tied with a single chromic tie, stick-tie
fashion… [*Whereas before these ligaments created
the pelvic floor, with the cervix at its center, now the
ligaments are being severed, so each one becomes a
pedicle, or stalk, with raw ends exposed and tied off
with something that resembles a staple.*] Following
this, straight Kochers were placed at the level
of the cardinal ligaments and the pedicles were
created again with a sharp knife and these were
tied with a single stick tie. The ties also included
the uterine artery pedicle. [*The uterine artery
was severed and tied off, dramatically disrupting the
pathways of blood and energy flows to every part of
her body.*] The vaginal cuff was then created with
the placement of two Heaney clamps across the
cervix. The vagina was then entered and a wide
vaginal cuff was taken without difficulty leaving
adequate amount of vagina and the specimen
was removed from the field. [*What he refers to as
the specimen—the uterus and cervix—were removed,
and the vagina was sewn together at the top into a
closed pocket where the cervix had been.*][34]

---

[34] Giuntoli, Robert, Surgical and Pathology Report from the hysterectomy performed
on Nora W. Coffey.

At the performance in St. Louis, the man who was with the woman who asked where the doctors were said, "The doctors aren't here to defend themselves because they know what they're doing is wrong." He talked about how a lot of doctors justify their actions with unscientific studies funded by drug or device manufacturers to spin their methodology to appear beneficial to women. "In other words," he said, "it's just a sales pitch to get you to buy their services. And what they sell are the same drugs and treatments advertised by the corporations that funded the study."

Many of the studies published in medical journals are based on the responses of 10 or 20 women (100 is exceptional). The studies are designed to prove a hypothesis formulated to promote a drug, a device, or a particular surgery. Follow the money. Thanks to recent media exposure, Americans are learning that the Food and Drug Administration (FDA) is little more than an arm of the medical industry. More and more doctors and medical industry executives are becoming politicians, like Senator Bill Frist, whose family owns the largest hospital chain in the U.S.[35] Most politicians accept large contributions from the medical industry into their campaign coffers, which amount to a quid pro quo. The president appoints the Surgeon General. FDA appointees who vote for or against drug and device approval are doctors, while their consumer advocate appointees don't have voting rights. Because of that, Nora declined FDA's suggestion to join a consumer advocate panel. It was a toothless tiger she wanted no part of. Drug and

---

[35] Freudenheim, Milt, "2 Largest Hospital Chains in U.S. Merge," *The New York Times,* October 3, 1993.

device manufacturers pay doctors to conduct and rubber-stamp their studies, and then they spoon-feed the results to FDA.[36]

By contrast, HERS relies on the experiences of women. The HERS Adverse Effects Data is the result of a detailed questionnaire where the responses of 1,000 women are reported verbatim. Their answers aren't altered or interpreted. There's no hypothesis to prove or disprove. It makes known what women report. The consequences of the surgery are so profound many women add several additional handwritten pages.

After Nora founded HERS, she did all she could to raise awareness...a dizzying pace she keeps up all these years later. Soon thereafter, she was interviewed in the local newspaper and on television. HERS received thousands of calls from the media exposure.

One of those calls was from a lawyer who saw Nora on TV. "Clearly she had great admiration for her client," Nora said, "and I offered to help in any way I could." Several days later the lawyer's client called Nora. "Joanne's words and thoughts were amazing, brilliant," Nora said of the woman. "She was able to lay out all the issues—the how and why of hysterectomy. And she did it in a clear, concise, but radical way." Nora and Joanne realized they could become a powerful team, and that was the beginning of a 23-year collaboration. "I felt like we knew each other immediately," Nora said, "like looking into a mirror. Here were two women, barely 90 pounds each, and barely five feet tall, but no one would describe us as small. Joanne was precise, and at times it drove me crazy," Nora continued, "because she frequently corrected my use

---

[36] Rosenberg, Martha, "What's Missing on Your FDA Drug Warning Label: Corporate Influence over the Safety Process," *AlterNet*, August 28, 2007.

of words. She always chose the most accurate language." As I listened to Nora tell me about meeting Joanne, I could relate to what she was saying, because Nora was the same way with me. If I talked about a woman who'd *had* a hysterectomy, Nora would correct me, saying, "She was *hysterectomized.* You have *dinner,* you don't *have* a hysterectomy."

"Joanne and I started working on a pamphlet," Nora said. "It was to be 'the white paper on hysterectomy,' as Joanne called it, which took two years to finish. Everything was carefully researched, every line discussed. The result is that every word in that pamphlet we're handing out at these protests is true for all time. If you're going to mean what you say," Nora said, "you'd better say what you mean."

Over time, Nora became more radical, but Joanne became less so. "Over time I guess we stepped into each other's shoes," Nora said. Together they made HERS what it is today—an independent, international women's health education organization whose work is mentioned in *Te Linde's Operative Gynecology* and, we've been told, is the subject of meetings and discussions at ACOG conferences. After a few public debates, one of which left a gynecologist so frustrated he was practically frothing at the mouth on television, no gynecologist will debate Nora.

Nora and Joanne worked together every day for over two decades educating the public. While HERS has helped millions of women avoid hysterectomy, gynecologists have hysterectomized more than 15 million more American women.

"Joanne is a woman who's incapable of living a lie," Nora said. "After the surgery, she immediately understood the profound, permanent changes caused by the removal of her uterus. She was strong, brilliant, and capable of doing just about anything she set her mind to before the surgery, but pretending that everything was okay after a doctor removed her female organs was something she couldn't do."

In the end, our small St. Louis audience walked with us out of the building as the lights were turned off behind us. It wasn't until then I noticed that the woman who asked the first question walked with a cane. We continued the conversation down the hallway and out onto the front steps…until finally we parted ways.

EIGHT

"Once missing, now identified."

Portland, Oregon—Nora W. Coffey

My children have fully supported me and my commitment to stop hysterectomy from becoming the legacy of another generation of women. Macy was seventeen years old, Jessica was seven, and Justin was just six when the surgery that devastated me also changed my children's lives forever. And although I tried to keep HERS separate from my home life, the needs of women all over the world soon made HERS a dominant presence in all of our lives. The fact that I was public about the effects of the surgery meant that my children could never pretend it wasn't so. When Jessica was eleven, she bought a scrapbook and filled it with interviews of me in newspapers and magazines.

I had protested for and against other issues when Jessica was little. She was a "flower child" dancing and singing to Joan Baez and Bob Dylan at be-ins, happenings, and boycotts, so it wasn't the protest itself in Portland that concerned me. Other than television interviews and the annual HERS conferences, when the Protest & Play tour arrived in Portland it would represent the first time that I'd be public about hysterectomy in her personal and professional territory. I'm a mother first and the president of HERS second. The last thing I wanted was for her to feel torn between supporting me and taking care of her own needs. It was *her* family that was fractured by what was done to her mother.

Jessica is well known and admired for her accomplishments. We welcomed publicity in every city, but here I had mixed feelings about it. I've always wanted my kids to be known for who they are, not for being the children of the woman who was in the news for founding an organization to stop other women from being damaged by doctors the way I was.

The protest was scheduled to take place at the Oregon Health Science University Hospital. Other protestors who were supposed to meet us called to say they were lost. Jessica and I couldn't find the main entrance to the hospital either, so Jessica waited outside to keep an eye out for the lost protestors as I went into the emergency entrance. The emergency wing was dimly lit and empty. I could hear a child crying somewhere, but there was no one at the in-take desk.

As I returned to join Jessica, we were greeted by the other protestors who had found their way. A security guard pulled up and said we had to leave. He was pleasant enough, but adamant. I wasn't concerned about what he felt we could or couldn't do, though, so I asked him to direct us to the main entrance.

"People don't walk to this hospital," he said. "You can't get in from the street. The entrance is on the ninth floor."

As we waited for him to explain, I thought, 'Now there's a concept. How much healthier would Americans be if all hospitals hid their main entrances, only allowing those with medical emergencies to enter? Death rates would plummet.'

The security guard explained that the only entrance was from the ninth floor of the parking garage, and there was in fact no public area to protest. So I asked him for suggestions of other hospitals with more pedestrian traffic. Relieved we'd soon be leaving, he made a few suggestions. Then Jessica told us about a hospital near where she used to work that sounded like a good fit.

The other protestors followed us to Good Samaritan Hospital, known to the locals as Good Sam's. Located in downtown Portland, there was plenty of pedestrian traffic, so we set up our materials and began handing out information.

Jessica's first employer in Portland had made generous contributions to HERS, and they continued to do so after Jessica moved on to another firm. I knew their offices were downtown, but it wasn't until I was standing on the street at the protest in view of their offices that I began to realize this could be a difficult situation for her. I would soon be carrying a sign that said "STOP Castrating Women NOW."

Jessica's quiet and laid back. Protesting in public was probably not something she would've considered doing under other circumstances. But the way she approached the protest wasn't unlike the way other daughters did. She helped carry the boxes but didn't immediately pick up a sign.

We had a good turnout, and Jessica watched as we staked out our spots. She stayed close and chatted when I wasn't talking with the public or walking out to cars that stopped for information. Before long, though, Jessica began offering pamphlets to people walking by.

A few doctors stopped by to find out why we were out there and to engage in the issues with us. For the most part they were supportive, reading the information we gave them as they walked away. Quite a number of nurses took the information, but several wouldn't take a pamphlet and made nasty comments. One nurse who was heading home after work said tiredly, "I had a hysterectomy." And then, after she paused to look at the materials we handed her, she said, "It's really good you're doing this. Thank you."

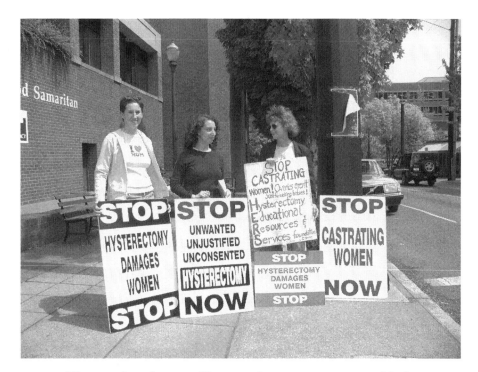

The pedestrian traffic was heavy, so we couldn't get to everyone passing by. Many of them patiently waited their turn. Some even returned the next day to thank us, which is something we hadn't experienced in other cities.

One man took the information from me, read it as he walked away, and then shortly thereafter he returned, asking if we accepted donations. He gave me his business card and handed me a $20 bill, saying, "Most people only talk about what's wrong with the world. They don't *do* anything about it."

Another man wanted to know in what ways hysterectomy damages women, as the sign that I was carrying claimed. I gave him a pamphlet, and he said, "My wife had the surgery." He then looked down the street, saying, "She died." And after a pause, he added, "She was very young." He then slowly walked away, reading the pamphlet. A few years later an article titled "The Case of a Woman Missing Since 2001 is Solved" appeared in *The Oregonian*, and I thought of the man I spoke with on the street in Portland when I read it:

> …It looked like a classic unsolved case: the body of an unidentified woman found floating in the Willamette River behind OMSI last December. Few clues. Leads ran out. Months went by, and no one claimed her. Then an envelope with two photographs and a short note arrived at the Multnomah County Sheriff's Office in April. "Detective Keith Krafve: Barbara Schmunk is the brunette on the left in both photos." That's all it said. But that was enough. DNA match this week confirmed that the body belonged to Schmunk, who disappeared in November 2001. The first key to solving the case was the profile. A deputy state medical examiner and a forensic anthropologist determined that the woman was 45 to 55 and stood 5-foot-5 to 5-foot-11. She'd had a hysterectomy, and she was wearing pantyhose and a body briefer. An article published in The Oregonian in March detailed the case. David Schmunk read the article. A few weeks later, he mailed the note and the photos of his wife taken the night she disappeared. Krafve talked to Schmunk, who had reported his wife missing Nov. 17, 2001. The same night, a 9-1-1 caller reported a woman jumping off the Ross Island Bridge. Police found a woman's glasses, cane and shoes on the bridge. A police dive team searched but found nothing. Barbara Schmunk, who was 45, matched the profile… But he needed a DNA match to close the case… Susan Hormann, the crime lab's DNA supervisor, was able to extract the DNA she needed. Hormann completed the comparison Thursday, and Krafve told Barbara

> Schmunk's family members, who declined to comment. Case closed.[37]

Case closed, indeed. I wonder how many people who read the article skimmed right past the clue Barbara Schmunk left behind on the bridge—a cane.

I help a lot of women through difficult times, but I understand when a woman can't bear the pain of living with what was done to them.

Two politicking, hand-shaking, baby-kissing state senators stopped by the protest to ask questions. They seemed interested and wanted to know more.

No wonder my daughter chose this city as her home. Some cities radiate a palpable anger, but I saw almost none of that in Portland. I counsel many women in Oregon, but only a few in Portland, where hysterectomy isn't an overt problem like it is in outlying areas and smaller towns. And yet, a large number of women approached us who said, "Thank you, but it's too late for me," or, "Why weren't you out here five years ago when I had mine? I never would've done it."

I didn't know hysterectomy and castration was a damaging surgery either, until it was done to me. Even if women who suffered from the adverse effects had told me, I don't know if I would've been able to fully understand what it meant or to realize that they represented millions of women whose problems were typical and common. I probably would've thought only a lobotomy could take my identity away from me. I was strong, healthy, highly sexual, vibrant, and not given to depression. I was educated, upper middle class, a musician, an artist, and an athlete. I had three children. All

[37] Green, Ashbel S., "The Case of a Woman Missing Since 2001 is Solved," *The Oregonian*, May 16, 2008.

that couldn't be taken from me by a routine surgery, or everyone would be talking about it. But now I know. Even after speaking with and emailing hundreds of thousands of women, it's my own experience that informs me most.

The same is true for the children of hysterectomized women. They don't need to read our materials to know that hysterectomy damages women. They know. In my family we rarely talk about it. We don't need to—it's understood.

NINE

Nerve damage.

Baltimore, Maryland—Rick Schweikert

The first person I handed a pamphlet to at Johns Hopkins University Hospital was a doctor who said, "Oh, just f___ off, would you?" A man and a woman walked closely behind him. When they heard him swear at me they stopped, watching the doctor walk away. They shook their heads and shrugged their shoulders, as if apologizing for him. They then took a pamphlet from me, and followed the doctor inside.

Johns Hopkins' website advertises that it's consistently rated "number one" by *U.S. News & World Report*, but Johns Hopkins is number one to us for a different reason. There would be a few close seconds, but they win the Gold for being the most arrogant, ignorant, disrespectful, and angry hospital faculty and staff we encountered in the 51 cities along the Protest & Play tour. Those aren't adjectives I'd want to use to describe the people caring for my family.

The main staging area for the protest was directly in front of the Pathology Department, a coincidence that wasn't lost on the protestors. One of them suggested that her uterus might be in there inside a jar of formaldehyde, like a trophy on a shelf.

Many of the protestors in Baltimore were hysterectomized at Johns Hopkins. It's a hospital where hysterectomy and the "language of surgery," as it was referred to in *The JHU Gazette*,[38] is taught to gynecology students. As of this writing, under the banner

---

[38] Sneiderman, Phil, "Unraveling 'Language of Surgery,'" *The JHU Gazette*, Vol. 36 No. 8.

"GYN/OB RESIDENCY AND FELLOWSHIP PROGRAMS," the Johns Hopkins website lists the following average statistics for their residents:

Procedure	Mean
Spontaneous Vaginal Delivery	383
C-Section	293
Forceps & Vacuum Delivery	73
TAH [total abdominal hysterectomy]	155
Vaginal Hysterectomy	53
Laparoscopy	132

With 293 C-Sections performed by the average medical student for every 383 natural births, it's no wonder the C-Section rate is rising in the U.S. But what's even more disturbing is that one hysterectomy is performed for nearly every two natural births. [39]

As I compose this chapter, one of the ad campaigns on Johns Hopkins website asks, "What if Ella Fitzgerald lived a few years longer? How much more could we dance? What if Ingrid Bergman survived cancer? How much more could we be inspired?" The women who protested with us in Baltimore might've asked, "What if a gynecologist had left me intact? How much better would my life be? How much better of a mother, a daughter, a friend, an artist, a musician, an athlete, an entrepreneur, an employee, a neighbor would I be?"

Since first meeting Nora and committing myself to helping her educate the public, I have had more questions than answers. How did we get to the point where doctors are able to convince millions of women they're better off without their sex organs? One

[39] "The Department of Gynecology and Obstetrics, GYN/OB Residency Program," Johns Hopkins, http://womenshealth.jhmi.edu/residency_mfm_programs/residents_visitors/training.html#benefits.

explanation is that doctors refuse to refer to the uterus and ovaries as sex organs. To quote Robert Mendelsohn, a Professor of Medicine at the University of Illinois, another reason is that doctors have attained a status in our lives that matches that of religious leaders. He compares hospitals to churches, doctors to priests, and birth certificates to baptismal records:

> I believe that more than ninety percent of Modern Medicine could disappear from the face of the earth—doctors, hospitals, drugs, and equipment—and the effect upon our health would be immediate and beneficial... For the hospital is the temple of the Church of Modern Medicine and thus the most dangerous place upon earth... There is plenty to be afraid of. The God that resides in the Temple of Modern Medicine is Death.[40]

One of the Baltimore protestors was a physician's assistant who was hysterectomized at Johns Hopkins. She was deeply religious, but neither the hospital's reputation nor the reputation of the colleague she put her faith in protected her. When she embarked on a personal crusade to tell her story, it fell on deaf ears within the medical community. That didn't stop her from engaging with even the most arrogant doctors during our protest with her daughter at her side.

One of the protestors I spoke with said she wouldn't have missed the Baltimore protest for anything, but she couldn't attend the reading of *un becoming* that night because it would be too painful for her. She did purchase the script from the HERS website, though, and after reading it she emailed to say she'd come to a performance in conjunction with the final protest in Washington, D.C., ten months later. She's now seen the play three more times since then.

---

[40] Mendelsohn, Robert, *Confessions Of A Medical Heretic*, McGraw-Hill, 1990.

There were two readings of *un becoming* to coincide with the Baltimore protest. The first was in Washington on Saturday at the 1409 Playbill Café, a small stage in the rear of a restaurant/bar. It was the first performance in a bar, and it was the first performance with a hysterectomized woman in the cast. Her daughter played the role of the child of a hysterectomized character in the play. As Nora said, they required no direction.

There were also two doctors in the reading, which was another first. One was a physician and the other was a specialist in child sleep psychology. They both said the play realistically portrayed the arrogance of the doctors they worked with.

In the talkback someone asked, "So are you doctors?"

"No, we're not," Nora answered. "Most of what I know about hysterectomy didn't come from books and medical journals. Rick's play matches what I know about hysterectomy and what most of the women I counsel say about their experiences."

The next day at the protest a doctor actually held up his hand to shield his eyes from our signs, but he couldn't help but notice our little mascot. One of the Baltimore protestors showed up with her lap dog, which she had donned with a homemade t-shirt that said, "Stop! Hysterectomy Damages Women!" When he read the dog's t-shirt he said, "Oh, give me a break!" I offered him a pamphlet, and he said, "I don't need that."

"Are you a gynecologist?" I asked.

He finally stopped, made eye contact for the first time, saying, "Yes, I'm a gynecologist, so I know!" before walking on again.

The second reading was on Sunday in Baltimore, by the Run Of The Mill Theater company. In the talkback someone commented that she thought the play was "a bit over the top," while another woman disagreed with her, saying she thought the play was understated. The second woman was "a registered nurse at a local hospital." Based on her experience, she said, "Gynecologists do whatever they have to do to get women onto operating tables. It doesn't usually have anything to do with medical problems."

It's not a coincidence that in the cities where we got the worst treatment from gynecologists we were the most welcomed by the public. The anger doctors directed at us was matched by the anger that was directed back at them from the people we spoke with on the street. One reason that gynecologists are angry with our message is they don't want women to be informed about the anatomical facts. For a gynecologist to acknowledge the effects of the surgery would be an admission that they do this to women with malice and forethought. At Johns Hopkins, that fact became plain as day. It was obvious in their anger and their arrogance.

"How do they sleep at night?" one protestor asked.

"By turning a deaf ear and a blind eye," Nora replied. Nora's parting shot to the next gynecologist was, "See no evil, hear no evil, know no evil?"

"It never hurts to read," I said to many of the doctors there. One of them stopped and replied, "You know what? You're right." He was a rare exception who stood there reading the pamphlet cover-to-cover. He then said, "Thanks. You're doing a good thing. I'm running late. Have a nice day."

"Well, there's one in a row," I said to Nora.

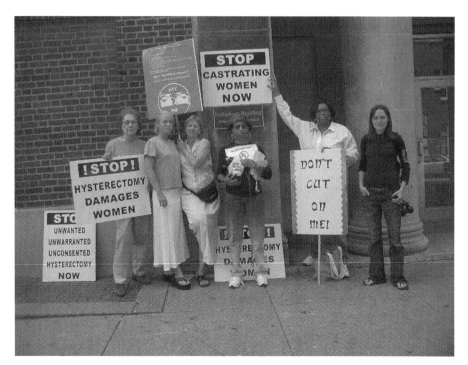

Our base station was near a busy bus stop. Passengers getting on and off took a pamphlet from us, and the bus drivers did too. A few of the drivers invited Eunita and Nora on board. As one of the buses pulled away, I could see the passengers with their heads bowed, reading the pamphlets.

More than any other city, in Baltimore we saw large numbers of women walking with a cane, a walker, or being pushed along in a wheelchair. Most were far too young to be having trouble walking. They may have been long-distance runners, body builders, manual laborers, mountain climbers, or just physically active in their families and communities before the surgery, but after their female organs are removed many women can't even walk without help. The first one I saw was a woman wearing a housedress and walking with a quad cane. I noticed her from two blocks away, and I don't think she took her eye off of us the whole way, stopping every twenty feet or so to rest. When she finally arrived at the protest site she held out her hands, took a pamphlet, and said, "God bless. I wish you would've been here before I had mine."

Many of these women had femoral neuropathy—damage to the femoral nerves in the leg causing pain and a loss of sensation. The neuropathy can be detected with an electromyogram (EMG). EMGs are used to test the function of nerve pathways to the muscles. Although the EMG may diagnose it, doctors rarely acknowledge that the neuropathy is the result of damage done during the surgery.

When women call HERS, Nora can only tell them the facts. In the case of femoral neuropathy, sometimes the nerve will regenerate, but it may not, and there's no way to make it happen—no drug, no surgery, no treatment can speed it up. If the nerve regenerates, it'll do so at the rate of about one to one and a half inches per year, so even if it does improve it might take decades. And that's just one of the many adverse effects that hysterectomized women live with. Here's a sampling of the thousands of emails HERS receives from women with femoral neuropathy (names omitted for confidentiality):

> My husband has said I changed after the hysterectomy but I'd never realized all the similar symptoms from chart 4. Following lists them: personality change, difficulty socializing, irritability, loss of energy, loss of sexual desire, loss of nipple sensation, diminished lubrication and that which has been bought and used has caused excessive burning and irritation, pain with intercourse, deep vaginal pain, suicidal thoughts, loss of short term memory, muscle aches, bone and joint pain, back pain, stiffness, pain that runs down buttocks and back of legs, tingling

and burning in feet usually in the evenings. Ok, so now I know the majority of women have similar symptoms; what can I do about them. My mother had breast cancer so I don't take HRT. What can I do? I'd greatly appreciate any help!

———

When I first woke up from the surgery I couldn't move my foot or leg. And they were very painful to the touch. I had a catheter for several weeks. I was in the hospital for 10 days. After that I started using a brace and a walker. I have damage to the femoral nerve, the tibial nerve, and the seral nerve. I can't be on my feet too long because my foot, ankle, and back hurt.

———

One year after the surgery, I have been suffering in a way I never imagine. I have been in constant pain, numbness, in my hands arms and legs. Pain in every part of my body! I have lost all of my sick days and vacation day due to getting sick. it's driving me crazy what am I to do or go about this? one thing is for sure, the doctor never told me of the negative side of this surgery except, "once it's done you can't retrieve it or go back; he promised I would be brand new!!!!!!!!! I am emotional mess. I am 41 years old married with children. it's not fair to the either. please help me with proper information or steps I should take. I am so unhappy at this time. I thought I be brand new enjoying life , my husband and my children!!!!!

———

I had a hysterectomy over a year ago since then I have no energy, am incontinent, stay to myself have very bad lower back pain , gained 40 lbs, and my feet hurt and crack to the point I almost can't walk. I saw a doctor and he said I had all the symptoms of depression and put me on antidepressants. I would not take them at first but he said when your depressed pain is worse. So I took them ,I did not feel any better ,except my back pain eased up. I felt like I had no emotions on those pills and all my life I was a happy person not depressed ,ever. I refuse to take them anymore. I know my symptoms were from the surgery, I had a complete hysterectomy at age 48 due to fibroids, a tumor ,and cysts. Now I feel like I am on my last leg and I am only 49. Please tell me how I can feel better and enjoy my life again and my job. I took hormones for a short time they really did not help me either. I saw this page and realized that other women had the same problems from having a hysterectomy. Who do I go to for help now, who will listen ? I am so tired of feeling tired . I used to work all day, come home work in my yard, clean my house and now I cry because I cannot do those things. Please give me some advice.

———

I have severe nerve problems in my legs and neuropathy in my feet. More pain in the right leg and foot than the left, but also some pain on the left. My feet are freezing or on fire and feel like a tight band is squeezing them.

Nora told me about a woman she counseled whose leg collapsed under her while carrying her baby down the stairs. No one was seriously hurt in the fall, but after that she stayed in bed and her husband hired someone to care for her and their two children. She committed suicide a few weeks later.

Many women who came out to the protest after seeing something about it in the newspaper asked, "Who's in charge?" or "Is Nora Coffey here?" We'd point out Nora to them, and they'd immediately begin asking questions, like, "What hormones should

I take to get better? I can't seem to find the right balance. I guess I'm a problem patient…what's the right combination to make me feel okay again?" I could see the pain on Nora's face as she told them the truth, that the loss is permanent, hormone replacement therapy is an oxymoron, and there's little to be done about it. No cure exists, and they would never be who they were before. A lot of them said, "But I just read about this natural hormone, and it says—"

"I wish I could tell you otherwise," Nora would say. "The damage can't be undone. There's no repair or drug that'll make you feel the way you did before the surgery."

Understandably, many women get angry hearing this. At first I'd watch Nora as she spoke with them, to make sure none of them took their anger out on her, but it was just the opposite. Although they sought a remedy, most of them already knew one didn't exist. They were thankful someone was honest with them. What they wanted was the plain truth, so they could end their futile quest for the remedy that would make them feel like the person they were before their female organs were removed.

TEN

An oasis from hysterectomy.

Boise, Idaho—Nora W. Coffey

I didn't want to leave Jackson, Mississippi because I could see how desperately women needed information about hysterectomy there. I hated to leave Boise because it's the only city where I felt women weren't in jeopardy...they weren't at risk.

I didn't realize such a place existed. It was surreal in the most wonderful way. The exhausted, angry women we met in Jackson simply didn't seem to exist in Boise. I didn't notice any women who, out of pain and profound fatigue, slowly lowered themselves into a seat. Instead, here women seemed to be walking naturally. When they stopped to talk with me it was about their lives, not their losses.

And yet, having counseled women in every state and from many countries around the world, I know that every woman with a uterus is vulnerable. In a city where almost every woman still has her uterus, in a country where the laws protect doctors and limit a woman's ability to seek damages, would Boise be able to remain a city unmarred by hysterectomy?

On the tiny plane to this charming city, I sat next to a woman who had moved away from Boise. Later, she returned because, as she said, "I love it so much." She then asked why I was visiting. Up to that moment she was talkative and friendly, but she suddenly got quiet when I told her about the protest.

Her sister was a nurse who, she said, "Was never the same after that."

"More hysterectomy scars are worn by the wives of doctors than anyone else," I told her. "Second are nurses."

The details of how her sister was bullied into surgery were unique, but the result was the same. Her sister lived in a small town in rural Idaho. After the surgery no one in her family wanted to talk about it. Her life was changed forever. She was still surrounded by family, friends, and the familiar peaks and valleys of the Rocky Mountains, but now she was profoundly isolated.

Maybe it was because of that conversation on the plane that I arrived in Boise prepared to find another Jackson, but it was just the opposite.

The hysterectomy anomaly in Boise might be due in part to the sparse population—if gynecologists hysterectomized all these women, I thought, what could they do next? But other isolated cities we'd visit, like Cheyenne, seemed to have high hysterectomy rates. Maybe women in Boise don't go to gynecologists as frequently as they do in Cheyenne. In Italy the hysterectomy rate overall is much lower than in the U.S. Umberto Cornelli, a doctor I interviewed in Milan, said hysterectomy is almost non-existent there because Italian women don't go to doctors unless they have life-threatening symptoms, while according to the Central Intelligence Agency women in Italy live three years longer than women in the U.S. Nicholas Bakalar of the *New York Times* writes:

> The study, published Monday in the online journal PLoS, analyzed life expectancy in all 3,141 counties in the United States from 1961 to 1999, the latest year for which complete data have been released by the National Center for Health Statistics. Although life span has generally increased since 1961, the authors reported, it began to level off or even decline in

the 1980s for 4 percent of men and 19 percent of women.[41]

The best thing about Boise from my perspective was that women there didn't need HERS like they do elsewhere. I hoped the materials I left behind on restaurant tables, park benches, and slipped between the pages of books in stores would be read out of curiosity…not need.

---

[41] Nicholas Bakalar, "Life Expectancy Is Declining in Some Pockets of the Country," *New York Times*, April 22, 2008.

ELEVEN

"The best thing I ever did."

Des Moines, Iowa—Rick Schweikert

> We see people as numbers, not patients. It's
> easier to make a decision. Just like Ford, we're
> a mass-production medical assembly line, and
> there is no room for the human equation in our
> bottom line. Profits are king.

This quote appeared in the *Des Moines Business Record*, where Malcolm Berko quotes "a prominent HMO executive" who, he says, is "a compassionate and generous man in his community... but at the office he turns into a blood-sucking Scrooge." The insurance executive, Berko says in the article, actually gave him permission to publish this shocking admission about America's medical assembly lines, where profits are clearly a higher priority than healing.[42]

I did my best to schedule the readings of *un becoming* around holidays, but the Seattle reading fell on Easter weekend, Des Moines on Memorial Day weekend, Philadelphia on Hallow-een weekend, and Los Angeles on the Winter Solstice, between Chanukah and Christmas. "But the good news about holidays and weekends," Nora said, "is that no hysterectomies are performed. I almost never hear from women who were hysterectomized over the weekend and never on a holiday, because hysterectomy is almost never an emergency. Very nice of gynecologists to take a break

---

[42] Malcolm Berko, "The real story about HMOs," *Des Moines Business Record*, September 2, 1996.

from hysterectomizing women to spend some quality time with their wives and daughters, don't you think?"

A woman is hysterectomized in the U.S. every minute of every hour of every day…but that includes weekends and holidays. When you break it down into banker's hours, another woman is hysterectomized every 10 or 15 seconds. So every weekend and whenever a holiday falls on a weekday, thousands of women in America wake up with their female organs intact who wouldn't if it was a regular workday. Insurance companies and Medicaid/Medicare save tens of millions of dollars on weekends and holidays, because they don't have to pay for unnecessary surgeries when gynecologists aren't working. So if profits are king at America's insurance companies, why is it they pay for so many medically unwarranted surgeries? Many people have tried to explain this to me, but I still have more questions than answers.

The Mercy Medical Center in Des Moines turned out to be a poor location for a protest, so we took it to the neighborhoods, handing out hundreds of pamphlets and play flyers. The Des Moines Register published a full-page story titled "Group to protest 'unwanted' hysterectomies" with a photo of the Baltimore protest. The reading of *un becoming* was also listed in every media outlet we could find, along with being listed as an "Iowa Top 10 Cool Things To Do This Week." In spite of it falling on a holiday weekend, the reading at the Kinkajou Coffee shop was standing room only.

Afterwards, a woman sitting to our left said she was "flabbergasted" by the play, because, she said, "I had a hysterectomy, and it was the best thing I ever did."

Nora said, "I don't know if you really mean to say that having your female organs removed is the best thing you've ever done, but it's my responsibility to tell the facts about what happens to every woman who undergoes a hysterectomy." Nora then spoke in detail about how surgeons go about removing the uterus from a woman's body.

A woman on the other side of the audience toward the rear talked about her life since the surgery. She addressed the other woman directly, but was respectful in a way that maybe only another hysterectomized woman could be. She understood why some women don't relate the problems they're having with the surgery itself.

There was a small group of women sitting near the owner of a metaphysical bookstore where we dropped off some pamphlets the day before, and they were also vocal. In the end, with little guidance from us, the audience brought all of the major points of discussion out into the open.

Even hysterectomized women have a hard time reconciling the aftermath of the surgery, given the dearth of basic information about female anatomy out there. Especially when hospitals say things like, "If a woman had good sexual function before the surgery, she will continue to have good sexual function afterward," as the Mercy Medical Center website claims. Surely Mercy doesn't mean to say they believe that sexual function after sex organs are removed depends on sexual function before the sex organs are removed. If so, do they also believe that if you walked well before having your legs amputated, you will continue to walk well afterwards?

TWELVE

Endometriosis.

Indianapolis, Indiana—Nora W. Coffey

Wishard Memorial Hospital is a suburban hospital, off the beaten track, down a long road, in a wooded area that was out of the reach of anyone who might have difficulty walking the considerable distance from the bus stop. It's increasingly common for hospitals to be built in remote areas, so it's not surprising that Richard Pérez-Peña of the *New York Times* reports the following:

> "I think the [ambulance] market was always there" but not exploited, said Dr. Daniel E. Weiner, chairman of the emergency department at St. Luke's-Roosevelt Hospital Center. He said the hospital had changed its view of ambulance services and emergency rooms, once seen as expensive burdens. "Now we think of the E.R. as the front door to the hospital, the big generator of admissions."[43]

At Wishard cars slowed down as drivers read our signs, nothing urgent at all about their appointments as they approached the entrance to the hospital. Putting a HERS pamphlet into anyone's hands is gratifying, but handing materials to a woman arriving at the hospital for an unwarranted surgery was especially satisfying. Some of them literally grabbed the steering wheel from the driver, forcing them to pull over.

Many women who are scheduled for surgery call HERS in the eleventh hour, frantically searching for information about hysterectomy because their intuition tells them something's not

---

[43] Richard Pérez-Peña, "Not Counting on 911, Companies Hire Private Ambulances," *New York Times*, July 6, 2003.

right with this picture. "Everyone seems to be rushing me toward a surgery," they tell me, "but I've got a bad feeling about it."

As one woman in Indianapolis reminded me, many of the women who don't find HERS until it's too late share a similar recurring fantasy. She said she relives over and over again the last moments before an anesthesiologist put a needle into her arm. Rather than slipping under and losing control, in this fantasy she gets up off the table and runs from the operating room, finds HERS, and continues to live her life intact, the person she was before the anesthesiologist's mask was put over her mouth.

I've been on the phone with women who called me from the hospital just before it was too late. They were watching television from a hospital bed when they happened to see me on a talk show or on the news and called the number I give out during interviews. Others were given our number by a nurse, something that has occurred more and more frequently as conscientious nurses and doctors who are disgusted by what gynecology is doing take matters into their own hands.

I'm able to talk with these women just moments before the surgery to give them the information their gynecologists have denied them. There have been many women who I literally talked out the revolving door of the hospital wearing nothing but a gown and slippers. They stay on the phone with me, telling me not to hang up as they leave the hospital, living in real time a fantasy that the rest of us can only dream of. *Before* it's too late.

On the opposite side of this remote hospital was a large parking garage. We stood just outside the doors of the main entrance facing an island plaza with benches between the two lanes of the boulevard driveway. Business must've been brisk, because there were throngs of customers and visitors passing in and out of the main entrance.

At some point I noticed what appeared to be a separate entrance for hospital staff up a hill, so I went to see if I could get a few doctors to take our materials. But not one of them made any attempt to communicate with me. They ignored me as if they were briefed to stay clear of us. At every hospital except Johns Hopkins, there would be a few doctors who, if nothing else, were curious and said, "So, what's this about?" But not at Wishard—it was a sustained, total lack of response from doctors.

Before long, four Wishard representatives joined us. This was a first. Two women began handing out a form letter to everyone who passed by while two men, oddly, sat down on the sidewalk watching them. The letter they handed out was printed on Wishard letterhead and was titled "Wishard Health Services Comments Related To HERS Protest."[44] As they distributed the letter they told people, "We don't do unnecessary surgery or hysterectomy." Predictably, this drew a curious response from the people they spoke with. To every person we handed our pamphlets to, the Wishard representatives made sure to also give them one of their 'we-deny-everything' letters.

As with all of the protests, we were low key. In general, we said nothing except, "Here's some helpful information you might be interested in," or something to that effect. Some of them took a pamphlet, some didn't. But the Wishard representatives were accosting their customers. Many people took their propaganda, scanned it, dropped it on the ground, and then went out of their way to get a HERS pamphlet.

---

[44] "Wishard Health Services Comments Related to HERS Protest," letter distributed by Wishard representatives at the Indianapolis protest, June 5, 2004.

1001 West Tenth Street   PH 317-639-6671
Indianapolis, IN 46202

Wishard Health Services Comments Related to HERS Protest

June 5, 2004

Wishard Health Services is the site of a protest this week by members of HERS – Hysterectomy Educational Resources and Services – a non-profit health education organization based in Bala Cynwyd, PA. Wishard Health Services was told by the HERS president that it is not singling out Wishard as a hospital that performs unnecessary or inappropriate hysterectomies, but is merely the backdrop for staging the organization's protest of all Indianapolis hospitals that perform hysterectomies.

In 2003, 245 hysterectomies were performed at Wishard Memorial Hospital. "I believe that the number of hysterectomies performed at Wishard is likely one of the lowest of the hospitals in Indianapolis," said Marilyn F. Graham, M.D., chief of obstetrics and gynecology at Wishard Health Services and associate professor of OB/GYN at the IU School of Medicine. Physicians practicing at Wishard are faculty of the IU School of Medicine.

"In fact, hysterectomies are performed rarely – only when medically necessary and only upon the request of the patient," she said.

"Our physicians would always investigate all other options and discuss these with our patients prior to making a decision to perform a hysterectomy. There must be documented pathology, and we must have exhausted all other medical alternatives."

At Wishard, women are extensively counseled regarding all of the potential consequences of a hysterectomy. When patients sign a consent form for a hysterectomy, Wishard Health Services takes an additional step to show patients in writing on a separate consent form that a hysterectomy is a form of sterilization. "In this way, we ensure that women clearly understand the consequences of this surgery," said Dr. Graham.

"At Wishard Health Services, our resources are very limited. Therefore, it is extremely unlikely that the hospital would recommend performing any medical procedures that are not absolutely necessary."

Wishard does not perform hysterectomies as a method of birth control. In fact the healthcare organization has a very extensive family planning program. There are over 10,000 patients representing every socioeconomic category receiving family planning services at Wishard clinics located throughout the city.

The heart and science of health and healing

The key sentence is, "In fact, hysterectomies are performed rarely—only when medically necessary and only upon the request of the patient, " as if these women drove across town to sit down in an operating room with a menu, saying, "Hm, let's see. Why don't you give me one of those hysterectomies that will shorten my vagina and put an end to my sex life. And while you're at it, I'll have a castration too." The women we spoke with told us a different story.

Many of them said they were hysterectomized at Wishard and were given little or no prior information about alternatives and consequences, except that they wouldn't menstruate anymore and "hysterectomy is a form of sterilization," as the letter says. Many of the women we spoke with said they regretted not knowing enough to avoid surgery. Some of them went on to tell us, with Wishard representatives just a few steps away, all the problems they were having after the surgery that they didn't have before.

The presence of the hospital representatives became more than annoying, for both their customers and us. Before long they actually began stepping in front of us in an attempt to block us from giving information to people who wanted our pamphlets. Rather than engage in their juvenile behavior, we crossed the driveway to be away from them.

As with every protest, we spoke with a lot of women who were having trouble walking after hysterectomy. Their movements were labored and slow. In spite of their difficulties, they went out of their way and pushed past the Wishard representatives to speak with us, sitting down on the benches with a HERS pamphlet and letting us know they identified with the information they were reading.

After a half hour or so, the Wishard representatives came across the driveway to join us again. And this time they added more staff to their numbers. So, I got into motion. I figured if they were going to crowd me, I'd give them a workout. They repeatedly threatened to call the police, but the police never came.

At some point a tall woman who was barely able to walk approached me with a menacing look on her face. She said, "That's why I'm here! That's why I'm *back* here! That's what screwed me up! I keep coming back to get them to do something about this, but it's not getting any better." She stayed with me, reading the entire pamphlet out loud at my side. She said she was hysterectomized for endometriosis, but she was in more pain after the surgery than before.

Novelist Hilary Mantel writes, "If you skew the endocrine system, you lose the pathways to self." The narrator of *Giving Up The Ghost* believes that her surgery was necessary, but most women who were told they have endometriosis don't have their diagnosis confirmed by a pathologist.[45]

Endometriosis occurs when tissue from the endometrium (the lining of the uterus) migrates through the fallopian tubes, where it implants itself in the pelvis. The endometrial implants in the pelvis bleed during menstruation, causing pain during menses. It can also be caused by surgery, such as a C-Section or laparoscopy, when endometrial tissue becomes displaced when the uterus is cut into. Women are increasingly diagnosed with endometriosis as gynecologists perform more and more unnecessary, invasive treatments.

The first symptoms of endometriosis are severe menstrual cramps. The endometrial implants in the pelvis bleed during menstruation, causing pain during menses. A woman is told she has endometriosis and put on drugs to stop menstruation. Finally, the doctor performs a diagnostic laparoscopy—an examination using a laparoscope, a tube-shaped instrument inserted through the ab-

---

[45] Hilary Mantel, *Giving Up The Ghost*, Macmillan, 2003.

dominal wall allowing the doctor to view the internal organs. It's common after laparoscopy for doctors to tell women they have Stage 4 endometriosis: "It's all over your organs, your bladder, your bowel…it's everywhere." It's not long thereafter she's in an operating room being hysterectomized and castrated.

Typically, after the surgery doctors say, "It's the worst case I've ever seen." So women are grateful that the alleged problem was solved, but when they get the pathology report nine out of 10 times they discover they didn't have it. Sometimes it's not until they go from doctor to doctor searching for a solution to their post-hysterectomy problems that someone asks them why the hysterectomy was performed in the first place. It's then, or when they call HERS, that they learn there was no endometriosis in the pathology report. Their organs were normal.

The only objective and non-invasive way of diagnosing endometriosis is with an MRI (magnetic resonance imaging) of the pelvis.

When endometrial implants migrate into the wall of the uterus as opposed to migrating out of the pelvis, as is the case with endometriosis, the condition is called adenomyosis, or endometriosis interna. Like endometriosis, the only objective way to diagnose adenomyosis is with an MRI of the pelvis, and similar to endometriosis, 9 out of 10 times the post-operative report fails to confirm adenomyosis. Adenomyosis is rare in women who haven't had children, and symptoms include continuous very heavy menstrual flooding without large blood clots and pelvic and vaginal pressure that feels like the uterus is trying to push out through the vagina.

It's unnecessary and unadvisable to undergo exploratory laparoscopy to determine if you have either of these conditions.

Operating rooms are dangerous places, and if you can obtain a diagnosis with a non-invasive test or study, it's safer than being in an operating room. Also, the objective film from the MRI will demonstrate whether or not you have the condition, rather than relying on a doctor who *says* they saw endometrial implants.

When it does exist, acupuncture is often effective at reducing bleeding, pain, or pressure, but the permanent cure is naturally-occurring menopause. With the exception of acupuncture, the most conservative treatment options, including Danazol, birth control pills, and GnRH agonists (such as Lupron and Synarel) have serious side effects. None of them can be used for more than a few months at a time. Although taking out the uterus and ovaries may stop endometriosis from growing in women who don't take hormones, HERS has yet to hear from a woman who had the surgery for endometriosis who wouldn't take back her pain to regain the functions of her female organs and her health and wellbeing.

Our experience with the Wishard representatives made me think about those who work inside America's hospitals. Not just the gynecologists, but the entire hospital staff that supports and enables them. Only one physician accepted our materials, while one woman after another told us they wished HERS had been there before they were needlessly hysterectomized and castrated at Wishard. If those doctors really cared about the wellbeing of their customers, all they had to do was stop, watch, and listen to these women.

A young woman who had difficulty walking approached me outside the hospital. She was determined to go out of her way to tell me her experience. Her story was unique, but I knew how it would end before she even began—no two stories are the same, but the outcomes are disturbingly predictable. I knew she'd tell me how she was fooled into believing the surgery was urgent, that it was a matter of saving her from an undetected or future cancer. Her doctor had used the same lines that doctors across the country use to get women onto operating tables. She woke up from the surgery forever changed, and now no one understood what she was going through. In the end she thanked me for listening and apologized for not being able to join us. No matter how strong she might've felt about what was done to her, it wouldn't make her strong enough to join a protest. She now needed a cane to walk because she had no feeling in her right leg. She said seeing us out there at Wishard was the first confirmation of what she already knew to be true, what no one inside the hospital would validate for her.

If only Wishard Memorial Hospital's letter matched what we heard and saw. Nothing would please us more than for there to be no need for our work, but the information we provide is vital…even for the women for whom it's too late.

What we saw at Wishard was a lot of poor, broken women and a lot of arrogant, uncaring doctors and hospital representatives.

THIRTEEN

"It's not just a baby bag."

Cheyenne, Wyoming—Nora W. Coffey

In Cheyenne I was interviewed by Allison Fashek of the *Wyoming Tribune Eagle*. She asked good questions and understood the relationship between the business of medicine and the business of politics. She seemed genuinely interested in truthful, straightforward journalism and had no problem using anatomically correct words without embarrassment, or talking about the consequences of the surgery that made most people squirm. She sent out a photographer who was equally open, interested, and curious.

The next morning I sat at the counter of an espresso café, reading the newspaper. No matter how many times you see yourself in the news, it's always a jolt, especially when you're so many miles from home in a café filled with strangers reading the same paper. There in the *Tribune Eagle* was my photo with a caption under it that read, "It's not just a baby bag."[46]

As the barista made espresso drinks, she greeted each person coming through the door. The way she moved behind the bar was telling. Her waist and hips were wider and fuller than her upper body. In her laughter I sensed something unnatural and hollow.

As my body and my personality changed after I was hysterectomized and castrated, I began to notice things about women I might not have otherwise. The way they walked, the way they talked, whether they made eye contact or avoided looking into the

---

[46] Allison Fashek, "Hysterectomy Group To Protest," *Wyoming Tribune Eagle*, June 13, 2004.

eyes of the person they were speaking with. Things that were once spontaneous now required thought. The women I counsel say they sometimes have to remind themselves of routine and ordinary social norms, like saying hello, smiling, being pleasant. That inner struggle is now obvious to me. It wasn't long before I realized I could tell if a woman had been hysterectomized simply by watching the way she moved and interacted.

Most women say they live with constant physical pain, they have a loss of affect (a blunting of emotional response and a lack of expression), and they're not who they were before. This change in personality, coupled with physical pain, irritability, and memory loss make ordinary interaction an effort for these women as they struggle to appear "normal."

Dramatic changes occur within a woman's body after hysterectomy. The broad bands of uterine ligaments are severed. These ligaments provide structural integrity throughout the pelvis and attach to the sacrum in the lower back (uterosacral ligament). Consequently, hysterectomized women can't walk, sit, bend over, or even stand the same as they could before the surgery. Because the ovaries are rarely left intact, the compounded struggles of castrated women are apparent to an informed observer.

The barista came over to take my order, but my mind was elsewhere. Two months before the first protest in Alabama, Rick and I sat together in the 45th Street Theater watching a rehearsal of the dinner party scene of *un becoming*. During a break, I commented that the way Tami Dixon was playing the role of the hysterectomized character Halley Ridge didn't ring true. "She's too engaged," I said.

"Well, it is a dinner party scene after all," he said.

"But your character doesn't want to be there," I said. "She's there, but she's not there. I don't know any other way of saying it."

"She's there, but she's not there…" Rick repeated. "Yeah. That makes sense. But how do I turn that into an action Tami can work with?"

"Since her surgery, Halley drifts away and there's nothing she can do about it," I said. "She plays with the hem of the table-cloth. Then she remembers she's at a dinner party, so she sits up straight, makes an awkward comment. Not really present, she drifts away again, returns to playing with the hem on the tablecloth. She checks the time on her watch, looks around to make sure no one saw her checking the time. She's alone in a room full of people."

Pulling me back from my reminiscences, the barista leaned her elbow on the counter as she took my order. She glanced at the newspaper spread out before me. "That's you, isn't it?" she asked. "I had one of those," she said with a shrug of her shoulders, as if to tell me it was no big deal. Then she added, "Well I'm fine, and I don't have any problems." She glanced away across the long countertop strewn with newspapers. "I had tumors, and I had to have it." The expression on her face spoke more loudly than her nearly whispered words. She may not have correlated the problems she was having with the hysterectomy before she read the article, but I could sense that the article had helped her connect the dots.

She was all too aware of the consequences of hysterectomy, because she was living with them. Accepting that they were the result of an unwarranted surgery was something else…not an easy thing to come to terms with. And now here it was in the local newspaper, spread out over the counter of her café, being read by customers, family, and friends. Now they knew too. She quickly took my order and turned to wait on someone else, relieved to not have to talk about hysterectomy anymore.

That night I felt claustrophobic in my room at The Plains, a hotel that looked like the set of a Wild West film. I needed to be outside. So I headed out of town on the first road that led me into the hills. When I pulled over and got out of the car I could hear animals moving around in the brush, but I felt safe and restful. I slept there, under the stars.

In the morning I returned to the same café. I noticed a woman sitting at one of the tables who wasn't dressed like the other women there. She recognized me from the paper and said she wanted to talk. Although she was a midwife, she said, she knew little about the consequences of hysterectomy. In fact, almost everything she assumed about it was wrong. Although this may come as a surprise to some, this level of misinformation among midwives is common. In general, the midwives and masseuses and holistic healers I meet are open to information but woefully misinformed. But she was eager for accurate information, so she could pass it along to other women in Cheyenne.

The Cheyenne United Medical Center was set back from the street. Like Wishard, no one would be walking to this hospital. And there was little chance of approaching passing cars without disrupting traffic. As I drove around the city distributing pamphlets in public places, the impact of hysterectomy in Cheyenne was obvious. I saw a lot of women struggling to get in and out of cars, men telling their struggling wives to hurry up crossing the street. A lot of sad, faraway eyes.

I visited a historic museum in a former train depot, but there were few artifacts. I felt lost standing in that cavernous, sparse museum. I imagined a similar museum for hysterectomy, except this one would be a former hospital where women stood staring at the artifacts of gynecological destruction—an operating table, a knife, female organs in a jar. How barbaric this will all look some day when we look back at a time when tens of millions of women were hysterectomized and castrated.

FOURTEEN

The whole is more than the sum of its parts.

Milwaukee, Wisconsin—Rick Schweikert

The market's wide open for those who prey on women and girls. From 5,000 to 6,000 girls begin menstruating every day in the U.S.[47] As gynecologist Stanley West said, "With proper planning, our advisers suggested, each year of practice would produce a lucrative 'crop' of women ripe for hysterectomy."[48]

West's medical license was suspended by the New York Department of Health. This is a quote from a "Determination and Order" against West by the Administrative Review Board for Professional Medical Conduct:

> We suspend the Respondent's License for three years and stay the suspension for all but three months. We place the Respondent on probation for three years, with the added requirement that the Respondent receive pre-approval for all surgery.[49]

Women who read books by doctors speaking out against hysterectomy may assume it means the doctors are conservative in practice and skilled surgeons, but it's not necessarily so. Gynecologists learn to say what women want to hear, but it shouldn't be assumed to reflect what they actually do in the operating room, or what women need to know about the many functions of the uterus.

[47] Estimate: Average age=12. U.S. births in 2007 = 4,315,000. Female= 51.1%. U.S. Census Bureau.
[48] West, Stanley, *The Hysterectomy Hoax*, Next Decade, 2002.
[49] "Determination and Order," Administrative Review Board for Professional Medical Conduct, New York Department of Health, February 6, 2003.

Most women are taught that the functions of the uterus are related only to menstruation and pregnancy. But even those natural functions are treated as if they might become problematic without medical intervention. Many women who contact HERS haven't even been taught the basic facts of menstruation.

During menstruation, there's a periodic shedding of the endometrium (the inside layer that lines the uterus) through the cervix and out through the vagina. When menstruation ends, the endometrium begins to proliferate (build up and thicken) until it sheds with the next menstrual flow. Menstruation varies from woman to woman in duration and amount of flow, and it changes throughout a woman's life until menopause.

Like fertility, pregnancy, and childbirth, the natural process of menstruation has become stigmatized and medicalized. For example, doctors don't tend to inform women of the benefits of being pre-menstrual. A few days prior to menstruation, many women have higher energy levels, greater cognitive acuity, and they're more sexual.

Instead, women who go to doctors for wellness exams are usually asked if there are any changes in menstruation, or if they're experiencing any problems. If they say they have mood changes, headaches, irritability, or changes in menstrual flow, they're likely to be told they have premenstrual syndrome (PMS). "There's no need to suffer," doctors tell women with PMS, and they're often prescribed antidepressants or medications to suppress menstruation, such as birth control pills, which are sometimes prescribed to be taken continuously to stop menstruation. But most of the symptoms of PMS are common and part of the natural ebb and flow of hormones. They don't require treatment. Interfering with the natural ebb and flow of menstruation by stopping the cycle (chemically or surgically) alters the endocrine system.

Exercise and diet can play an important role in the amount of menstrual flow, PMS, and mood. Weight-bearing or aerobic exercise may help—jumping rope is particularly beneficial. Avoiding salt and dairy may help reduce premenstrual bloating. If you're prone to headaches, avoid caffeine. Raspberry tea reduces menstrual cramps, and black cohosh (a perennial plant that is part of the buttercup family) may reduce heavy menstrual bleeding.

The most effective way to decrease heavy menstrual bleeding is to lie on your back, elevate your feet, and put an icepack on your pelvis. It's common for women to use heat for menstrual cramps because it feels good, but heat actually increases the blood flow and the amount of menstrual bleeding.

Gynecologists often recommend dilation and curettage (D&C) for heavy or irregular bleeding, as well as for postmenopausal bleeding and polyps. If you have polyps, polypectomy uses a wire loop to remove polyps at their base and is an effective, less-invasive treatment. Most endometrial and cervical polyps are benign. If a D&C is performed for heavy bleeding caused by a submucosal fibroid, a D&C will worsen the bleeding. A risk of multiple D&Cs is Asherman's Syndrome, a painful condition caused by scar tissue and adhesions in the uterus, which can result in infertility and chronic pelvic pain.

The journal *Obstetrics & Gynecology* reports that diagnostic D&Cs fail to accurately diagnose a condition 10–25% of the time.[50] Perforation of the uterus during D&C is also a risk. Many doc-

---

[50] Word, G. and Gravlee, L.C. et al, "The fallacy of simple uterine curettage," *Obstetrics & Gynecology*, 1958; Grimes, D. A., "Diagnostic dilation and curettage: a reappraisal," *Obstetrics & Gynecology*, 1982.

tors concede that, "The incidence of perforation [of the uterus] is extremely difficult to establish; many operators refuse to admit that this complication has occurred…[resulting in] an immediate or remote threat of death."[51]

According to the Centers for Disease Control and Prevention, in 2005 there were almost 2,000,000 non-obstetric "operations on the female organs." Of those, 10,000 were performed on girls "under 15 years."[52] More than 5,000 women and girls under the age of 24 are hysterectomized each year.[53] HERS has learned from the millions of letters, emails, and phone calls over the last 25 years that, except for pregnancy and menstruation, women aren't informed about the functions of the female organs prior to surgery.

Wellness checkups for women are on the rise, and the average age at the time of hysterectomy in women who contact HERS is falling—a decade ago the average age was 42. Now it's only 36. The fastest growing age group of women who call HERS is teenagers who are told they need exploratory surgery. Most of the girls who call HERS say they never heard the word hysterectomy before a doctor removed their female organs…before they had a chance to enjoy being a woman. Some are so uninformed they email HERS after the surgery to ask if they can still get pregnant.

Our Wisconsin protest coincided with the National Women's Studies Association (NWSA) Conference, where Nora was an invited speaker. In addition to educating women about female

---

[51] W. A. R. Cooke, MD, "Perforation of the Uterus," *Canadian Medical Association Journal*, Volume 93, September 11, 1965.
[52] "Advance Data No. 385, United States 2005," *CDC*, July 12, 2007.
[53] National Hospital Discharge Survey, Hysterectomy Surveillance—United States, 1994—1999, *CDC*.

anatomy, it was an opportunity to draw attention to the Protest & Play year and to inspire other activists.

I was already in Milwaukee for a rehearsal at the Boulevard Ensemble Studio Theatre (B.E.S.T.) when I got a call from Nora. "My flight was cancelled," she said. "I'm snowed-in in Philly, so I won't be able to speak at the conference. You'll have to do it for me."

I've found talkbacks after readings of the play to be easier with smaller audiences. You get to the heart of the issues faster. In the same way, speaking to a small audience at the NWSA conference also had its advantages. But I was disappointed that hysterectomy, the most urgent issue facing American women today, was relegated to a small round-table discussion in a large auditorium that was being prepared for a plenary presentation titled "Feminist Uses Of Science and Technology."

Genevieve Carminati, the Women's Studies Coordinator at Montgomery College in Rockville, Maryland, spoke first about the impact of hysterectomy on the fabric of our culture. "This epidemic removal of sex organs," she said, "undermines women's health and minimizes their capabilities." I was the second panelist, focusing on hysterectomy statistics and exploring the reasons why the removal of the female organs flies below the radar of most women's organizations. The final panel was Megan Feifer and Emily Kane-Lee who spoke about "the magic and mystery of menstruation...to celebrate and embrace women's bodies and explore what consumer options and choices menstruating women can make in honor of their bodies and the environment."

Surprisingly, organizations you'd think might support our work, don't. For example, a representative of Planned Parenthood in Salt Lake City contacted HERS, saying, "For many of our

Mormon women here in Utah, hysterectomy is their only form of contraception." She then contacted the Planned Parenthood in Philadelphia, requesting they write a letter to HERS opposing hysterectomy informed consent legislation.

The NWSA, likewise, would seem to be another natural ally. But most of the women's studies academics we've spoken with are more focused on getting tenure and pursuing their own scholarship than providing practical knowledge to students. Several NWSA members named their support for a woman's right to choose as their reason for not supporting HERS, somehow confusing our opposition to unconsented hysterectomy with an opposition to abortion. And many women's studies scholars seem offended by the notion that the female organs are important to a woman's identity. They see a woman's identity as more cultural than biological. But what are we, if we're not defined by our bodily functions?

Women's Studies scholars should be interested in this subject because, if nothing else, it's something that can only be done to women. It has gender, social, political, and economic consequences. It malforms every aspect of the women directly affected—anatomically, physiologically, psychologically, professionally, socially, and economically. The unrestricted destruction of women's bodies and lives for over a century is a medical atrocity.

It's a wonder then that female anatomy and the functions of the female organs aren't part of the curriculum of every feminist academic and required reading for all women's studies students. What other issue impacts women more than hysterectomy? How is it that a discipline focused on women doesn't make available to every student the anatomical facts that define women as women?

While one in five women report being raped or sexually assaulted,[54] one out of every three is hysterectomized[55] without the information required for consent. Legally, unwanted touching, whether it's rape or unconsented surgery, is considered battery. Each year there are almost five times more women needlessly hysterectomized and castrated in this country than report being raped.[56] Rape is a criminal offense, while the unconsented removal of the female organs isn't a punishable crime.

A lot of Women's Studies students I've spoken with are surprised to learn that the Equal Rights Amendment failed. "Wait a minute," they say, "ERA passed, didn't it?"

"No," I answer them. "Our country failed to ratify the ERA." The legal doctrine that would give women equal rights lacked enough support to pass.

We received little response to the thousands of emails, letters, faxes, and phone calls we made to women's studies faculty and staff at more than 100 universities around the country regarding our Protest & Play year. That included our stop in Milwaukee, where our protest and reading of *un becoming* coincided with the NWSA conference. And when we did speak with women's studies faculty, their comments were confusing.

"Doctors don't do unnecessary hysterectomies anymore," they often said. "But they do," I'd say, noting that even ACOG acknowledges as much. "Well, it's not a good fit for us right now." Oth-

---

[54] Collins, Karen Scott et al, "Health Concerns Across a Woman's Lifespan: 1998 Survey of Women's Health," *The Commonwealth Fund*, May 1999.

[55] Larson, Nancy, "Experts: Two-thirds of hysterectomies unnecessary," *CNN,* March 3, 2008.

[56] "Every year approximately 132,000 women report that they have been victims of rape or attempted rape," National Organization of Women, http://www.now.org/issues/violence/stats.html. This is compared with 621,000 reported hysterectomies each year on average, according to the CDC.

ers would bring up the abortion issue, wrongly conflating our campaign with those who would eliminate a woman's right to choose. "We support a woman's right to choose," they'd say. This comment always stopped me cold, because hysterectomy has nothing to do with abortion. A few went so far as to tell me they were opposed to waiting periods for abortion, and compelling doctors to educate women prior to hysterectomy would set a bad precedent. Are there really feminists out there in favor of a woman's right to choose a surgery without being informed of its adverse effects?

"We have fought long and hard to get good healthcare for women. We need more healthcare, not less," I was told. But I (and many researchers) disagree with the assumption that more medicine means better health. Certainly you agree, I'd say, that hysterectomy without informed consent is bad for women's health. "These kids are teenagers. They don't care about hysterectomy," they said. "And we have people in our health clinic who teach our girls everything they need to know." But clearly, they aren't getting the job done, because we rarely meet a woman who understands female anatomy and the functions of the female organs.

That evening in Milwaukee, we dined at an old-world restaurant called Three Brother's, then took in a polka band at Art's Concertina Bar. The next day the Milwaukee protest began.

Grace, Larry, Bob, Sinora, and Sinora's four children joined Nora and me at the Froedtert Hospital. I had to leave early to sit in on a rehearsal of *un becoming* at B.E.S.T., but I only got a short distance away when I got a call. It was Nora asking if I had the protest permit.

I returned to the protest site to find police cars parked up and down the street. Across from where we set up our materials, Nora was talking with a cop who was more than twice her size. I handed him the permit, and he studied it a while before calling into the precinct. Just as I was preparing to leave again, he said, "Wait a minute. Your permit's no good. You can't issue a permit on private property."

"I researched the property lines myself," Nora said, "this is public property."

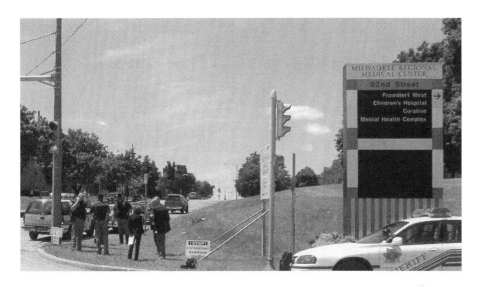

"No, it isn't," he said. "And this street is the boundary between the City of Milwaukee and the City of Wauwatosa. Your permit doesn't have jurisdiction here. If you continue protesting, we'll have to arrest you."

They left no doubt that if we continued they'd do just that. We were pretty much at the end of our protest day, so we decided to postpone the dispute, research the property lines back in our hotel room, and figure out what to do then.

The next morning, at 11:00 a.m. sharp, a Wauwatosa police car arrived at the protest. And another. And another. And the sheriff too. Just when we thought we were about to be arrested, the Milwaukee police also arrived on the scene. This came as a great relief,

because I figured all we'd have to do was show them the map we
downloaded from the City of Milwaukee website and the matter
would be resolved. Instead, the Milwaukee cop concurred with the
neighboring police, saying the map we found online was outdated.

"But it's from your website, and here's the permit that con-
forms to that map. If this isn't the right one, where is it?"

"It's down at the station," the Milwaukee cop said.

"Then let's go get it."

"I can't. It's bolted to the wall of the station," he said.

"Well, I guess we can all take a look at it together when you
arrest us."

He looked at Larry who was videotaping our entire
conversation. "I'm not the one who'll arrest you," he said. "It's
Wauwatosa."

"I'll tell you what. Give me the address of your police station, and I'll go take a look at the map," I said.

Finally he smiled and scratched the back of his neck. "I've
been doing this a long time," he said, "and I don't think you're
right. But why don't you let me go talk with these guys and see if
we can't come up with something."

"We'd appreciate that," I said. "This map says our permit's
legal, and we've called our attorney and the ACLU. We're prepared to be arrested, if that's the way it has to be."

"Okay," he said. "Just let me go down and talk with these
guys."

The police talked for a long time in one of the squad cars
while we continued handing out materials. Finally the Milwaukee
cop got out of the Wauwatosa car and approached us.

"You know what?" he said, glancing over at Larry, who continued videotaping. "It turns out you're right. You know what this is? This is a simple case of an honest misunderstanding. It turns out the map you have there is the right one. So you're okay."

He then became exceedingly friendly with us, walking away with one of our pamphlets in his hand. The Wauwatosa cop, however, waited until the Milwaukee cop was gone and threatened me menacingly that if we "so much as set a foot in the street and held up traffic" he'd arrest us.

The reading of *un becoming* that afternoon at B.E.S.T. was one of the better performances of the year. Under the direction of Marjorie Schoemann, Amy Callahan's performance of Halley Ridge was so poignant we considered flying her in to play that role in the production at the end of the year in Washington, DC.

There was an acting class at B.E.S.T. earlier in the day, and one of the actors decided to stay for the reading. She considered leaving because of the heat (it was a sweltering June afternoon and the theatre wasn't air-conditioned), but she stayed until the end, fanning herself continuously with the play program. She took part in the talkback, and was the last person to leave.

The next day, I was already on a plane returning home when dark clouds crept over the horizon. After two days of sunshine, the storm unleashed torrential rains. In spite of the storm, Grace, Nora, and a few others handed out a few more cases of materials. Nora was drenched head to toe and had to change her clothes in the rental car on the way to the airport…off to South Dakota.

FIFTEEN

The need for validation.

Rapid City, South Dakota—Nora W. Coffey

When I spotted a construction crane looming over the horizon, I knew I was close to the Rapid City protest site. I got everything set up as usual, and before long someone came out of the hospital with an urgent stride and an expression on his face that seemed to say, "Ma'am, I need to have a word with you!" As he crossed the street I steeled myself for the usual litany. But instead of threatening me, he extended his hand. "Hello," he said, "I'd like to welcome you to Rapid City and the Rapid City Regional Hospital." He then introduced himself, saying, "You're more than welcome to come inside to use the restroom or the cafeteria. Feel free to use the hospital's parking lot. Just please don't bring your signs or pamphlets inside the hospital. I've got two girls of my own at home," he said.

Our protest against unconsented hysterectomy was big news in Rapid City. I was interviewed for the *Rapid City Journal*. In the article, Helen Frederickson of Rapid City Regional Hospital claimed that hysterectomies performed there were medically warranted.[57] I'd like to review the hysterectomy pathology reports and informed consent process with Rapid City Regional or any hospital that would allow it.

Protesting in these smaller cities was particularly fulfilling. The medical center was often the major industry in town. I spoke with countless women who thought they were the only ones to experience the aftermath of hysterectomy and castration, until

---

[57] Harlan, Bill, "Hysterectomy Protest Set Here For Friday," *Rapid City Journal*, June 24, 2004.

the protest arrived there. In more rural areas we were far more likely to hear someone say, "My mom had one, and she's fine." But then, after a brief conversation, it became clear that Mom was anything but fine. In reality she was in poor health and a different person since the surgery. She simply couldn't talk about it, in a place where such things aren't mentioned.

Many vans and SUV's with elderly women passed by. A few of them stopped to get materials and tell me they saw me on the news and in the paper. They thanked me, saying, "Now you watch out for this traffic, dear."

The people of Rapid City were curious, friendly, and receptive. They seemed sincerely concerned about whether I was okay out there, and it was obvious that many of them understood the aftermath of hysterectomy from first-hand experience. They took pamphlets from me, but few stopped to talk about it. A struggling, hysterectomized woman has a well-kept secret in places like Rapid City. That silence is part of the problem.

When I returned to the historic Alex Johnson Hotel after the second day of the protest, the street was lined with Harley Davidson motorcycles. There was a Vietnam veteran bikers rally that weekend. A warm and sunny day, all the outdoor tables were filled, mostly with middle-aged men with tattoos up and down their arms. Initially they stared at me out of curiosity, reading the signs I carried, but then they looked away, avoiding eye contact.

Heading toward the hotel, I walked up to the center of the tables. Everyone fell silent. The hush was so obvious, I had to say something.

"So. Do any of you know what a hysterectomy is?" No one said a word. No one moved. "Well, let me tell you," I said, and I proceeded to give them a brief anatomy lesson.

They shifted in their chairs, they coughed and cleared their throats, but not one of them said a word. And not one of them got up to leave. When I finished speaking, I spotted a table with an empty chair beside a guy with a lot of tattoos sitting alone. I asked if I could sit down. He blushed all the way up to his receding hairline.

I propped up one of the signs against the window of the hotel and took a seat beside him. After a while, a woman came over, asking if she could take my picture. When she got the camera over her right eye, her left eye squinting, she said, "I had one of those," and then she snapped the picture. She held the camera there for a long time, but then finally she lowered the camera and set it on the table.

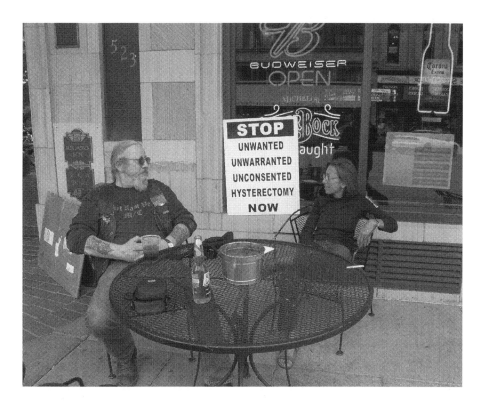

"Do you want to talk about it?" I asked.

"Nope," she said, and walked away.

That evening I headed out for dinner. Sitting there in my protest t-shirt, I read a book while eating an exceptional meal. I could feel a woman on the barstool beside me staring at me. She was pretty, blond, in her late 20s or early 30s. Her laughter sounded forced. Being social seemed like an effort. Her movements were unnatural and lacked spontaneity.

Although I wanted to speak with her, I avoided saying anything. Finally, though, our eyes met and she said hello. As her husband spoke to the bartender, she told me about her budding career as a young executive. I told her about HERS and the Protest & Play year.

Immediately her demeanor changed. It was like a switch had been flipped. Her muscles relaxed and her body language changed. As if someone had just pulled off her mask, she nervously told me she'd "had one" less than a year before. She smiled, as if to say she was getting along okay, and then turned to her husband, telling him enthusiastically, "This is Nora Coffey, the woman in the newspaper protesting at the hospital."

He looked anxiously at her, and then said more to me than her, "Oh come on, that's over! It's done and we're not talking about it anymore."

"No," she said after a moment, "I want to talk about it."

He moaned and quickly strode away from the bar. Alone now, we were able to talk more openly. She said the surgery was performed for endometriosis. I told her it's wrongly diagnosed nine times out of ten and that hysterectomy is never warranted for endometriosis.

She said little, but she was clearly bewildered by what the surgery had done to her body. She said she couldn't understand why she felt awkward talking to people since the surgery, both socially and at work, people she once communicated with so effortlessly. She asked what remedies might be out there for the variety of problems she was experiencing, saying, "I really wanted to have children."

For some reason I had no pamphlets that night, so I asked for her address, to send her materials in the mail. But just as she began to write it down for me, her husband returned from the restroom. This time he repeated himself more adamantly, saying, "We're *not* talking about this!" So now it was her turn to escape to the restroom.

Alone with him now, after a pause he began to speak. "You know, she's really had a hard time. And it's time for us to put this thing behind us. She's finally back at work, and beginning to do normal things. We just need to leave well enough alone."

"Maybe she doesn't want to leave well enough alone," I said. "Maybe she needs to know." When he didn't respond to this, I said, "I came here to have dinner, not talk about hysterectomy. But I wouldn't consider withholding information from her."

When she returned, we talked for a long time. Her husband sighed and paced nervously, repeatedly trying to get her to leave. The bartender was clearly anxious about our conversation. After a while, she said, "I can't tell you how grateful I am. I just feel so different. I didn't know what was happening to me, and I don't have anyone to talk to about it."

When the couple left, the bartender asked me about the conversation. I wouldn't share what she had told me in confidence, but he said he overheard bits and pieces. He was kind and had known the couple a long time.

He obviously cared about her. But there was something else. Because it had happened so many times before in so many other protest cities, I knew it was coming. When he got quiet, I could hear the words before he even said them: "My mom had a hysterectomy. When I was a kid."

"Speaking with your friend here was like opening a Pandora's box for her and her husband," I said. "It's a lot to accept, but now she knows hysterectomy wasn't the only option. Now she can help other women. Her husband needs to believe if they just act normal everything will *be* normal. But his need to shut it out and pretend that all's well denies her reality. She needs to talk about it. At least now she knows that what she's experiencing is real, she's not imagining it, and she's not losing her mind."

SIXTEEN

55 wrong opinions.

Hartford, Connecticut—Nora W. Coffey

While protesting in Hartford, I counseled a woman who called HERS after hearing from doctor after doctor that the problems she was experiencing were all in her head. She knew otherwise, but she was relieved to find validation. That relief, though, as is often the case, led to despair. "It isn't fair," she said. "How do doctors get away with this?"

She was right, of course, but after an hour of listening to her anguish I had to move her in another direction.

"I want you to do me a favor," I said. "After you get off the phone, I want you to go sit in front of a mirror and look yourself in the eye. I want you to decide whether you're going to spend your life lamenting what was done to you with no one there to hear you, or if you're going to get up out of your chair and tell the world so this won't be done to your daughter." After a pause, I said, "It's a choice. You have the power to change this for other women."

In response, she said, "I bought a gun."

What do you do when you can't change what's been done to you? Only a few choices remain. "I have considered every option," I told her. "The only thing that will mean anything will be to continue using every waking moment of my life to stop the Robert Giuntoli's of the world from doing this to other women. Right now I'm in Hartford, the 15th city on a 51-city protest tour, and there are a lot of women here who need this information."

Long before I arrived in Connecticut, I sent the gynecologists at Hartford Hospital information about the protest. I also sent it to Stephen Curry, the Director of Women's Services and the Chair of Obstetrics & Gynecology at the University of Connecticut. This was his emailed response:

> For some reason I received your schedule of protests that indicates you will be at Hartford Hospital in July. I am flabergasted in that in the 14 years I have been Director of OB/GYN at Hartford Hospital we have done everything possible to decrease the number of Hysterectomies. We have the largest uterine embolization program in the state. Please review our Web site. I could go on for several pages about our programs if you want. Why Us???

Here's what I emailed back:

> Dr. Curry,
> Thank you for your email. You have been on HERS mailing list since 1990, which explains why you received notice of HERS nationwide protest and all other HERS mailings for the past fourteen years.
> It is encouraging to know that in the past fourteen years you have "done everything possible to decrease the number of hysterectomies" performed at your hospital. However, until the number of unwarranted, unconsented (which includes hysterectomies performed on women who were not fully informed of the functions of their female organs and the consequences of surgically removing them), and unwanted hysterectomy is zero, it is not low enough.
> With regard to Hartford Hospital having the largest uterine embolization program in the state, it does not serve women well to trade one damaging surgery for another. I will send you some of the medical journal articles which document the damage caused by UAE.

> I would like to meet with you to discuss these is-
> sues when I am in Hartford the week of July 3rd.
> If you are interested please let me know of a con-
> venient time after 2 p.m. any day that week.
> Nora W. Coffey
> HERS Foundation

In response to my email reply, Curry scheduled an appointment to speak with me. When he called he asked if he could put
me on the speakerphone. He said there were several people with
him, and I asked them to introduce themselves—a gynecologist,
a public relations person, an attorney, and Curry. The PR person
did a lot of the talking at first, and then I asked them a range of
questions.

Curry began telling me about a hospital in Hartford he felt
was doing a lot of unnecessary hysterectomies, but he stopped mid-
sentence, as if he realized he shouldn't mention them by name.

I asked him what he tells women about the consequences
of hysterectomy when he recommends surgery. He said he and
everyone in his department spends an hour with each woman going over all the informed consent information. Again I asked him
what he tells them. He said he tells women they won't menstruate
and get pregnant after the surgery. Then he tried to change the
subject.

I returned to the subject of informed consent, asking him if
he tells women that removal of the ovaries is castration.

"No," he said, "that would be inflammatory."

But if he wanted women to be fully informed, I said,
wouldn't it be prudent to use the medically correct words? When
he didn't answer I told him I think it's wonderful that everyone
in his department spends an hour fully informing every woman

prior to undergoing a hysterectomy, so surely he wouldn't mind if I talked with them.

"Not at all," he said.

Someone in the room suggested that now I could see that they don't do unnecessary hysterectomies, so HERS didn't need to protest there. I told them I'd take everything they said into consideration, and after an awkward goodbye we hung up.

I visited their website to find contact information for Curry's 55 gynecologists, and the next day I began calling them. I introduced myself, saying, "I'm sure Steven Curry told you I'd be calling." Some of them said, no, some said Curry had called them to let them know I'd be calling, and others said he called a staff meeting to discuss the matter. I asked each one the same question I asked Curry, and each one adamantly told me they give full informed consent disclosure and spend about an hour in pre-hysterectomy consultation. But like Curry, none of them took more than a couple of minutes recounting what they tell women in that hour of consultation. I told each one of them I had an hour scheduled for each call, so they could take their time answering my question. But only two gynecologists gave more than the most basic information beyond cessation of menstruation and no longer being able to conceive. And although two of them did say some women notice a difference sexually, neither of them provided anything close to complete information.

When I told Rick about all this he asked for Curry's phone number, so he could hear it for himself. He called Curry and asked him several questions, to which Rick got similar responses to the ones Curry gave me. Curry then asked Rick what he knew about the functions of the organs and the consequences of the surgery.

So Rick told him…in great detail. Finally Curry interrupted Rick, saying, "That's just not true. I don't know what the HERS Foundation has been filling your head with, but my wife had the surgery and she's just fine."

Rick asked him if women can still experience uterine orgasms without a uterus, to which Curry replied that the uterus isn't a sex organ, and a lot of women don't have uterine orgasms *with* a uterus. Rick then asked him why, if women need a uterus to experience uterine orgasms, doesn't he consider the uterus a sex organ? Curry didn't respond.

A few weeks after these phone calls I arrived at the Hartford Hospital for our protest. WVIT, NBC Channel 30, stopped by the protest, and Nader Abu-Rabei interviewed me. A woman ran out of the hospital with a cell phone pressed to her ear. As she approached me she said, "You said you wouldn't come here!"

"No," I replied, "what I said is I'd take everything you said into consideration. I did just that, and I decided the Hartford Hospital was precisely the right place for us to stage a protest."

"But we told you we don't do unnecessary hysterectomies!" she said.

"Yes, I know. Why don't you go talk with that woman there across the street holding the sign that says 'STOP! HYSTERECTOMY DAMAGES WOMEN' and ask her if unnecessary hysterectomies are done at your hospital." I then pointed down the street in the other direction. "And that one over there carrying the 'STOP CASTRATING WOMEN NOW!' sign?" I said. "Ask her whether or not this hospital removes healthy ovaries from women. Both were operated on here."

The first protestor I pointed to crossed the street to join us. Finally the woman from PR put her phone in her pocket as the protestor told her what her life had been like since the surgery. The second protestor came over and did the same. Before long the woman from PR simply turned around, walked back inside the hospital, and didn't return.

No one did. Not Curry, or the attorney, or any of the other 55 gynecologists. We all got back to work. The woman from PR returned to spinning her hospital's reputation, and we returned to educating the public.

SEVENTEEN

The vote is mightier than the dollar.

Boston, Massachusetts—Rick Schweikert

Nora and I papered the Harvard campus with pamphlets and stacks of flyers for the Boston reading of *un becoming*, and then we got the protest underway at the Brigham and Women's Hospital, "A Teaching Affiliate of Harvard Medical School." The medical school was adjacent to the hospital, and there was also a lot of non-student pedestrian traffic, which made for an excellent protest location.

One of the protestors told me about the anger she felt when she woke up from exploratory surgery for benign fibroids. She said she was given no information about alternative treatments or adverse effects. When she understood that her life was permanently changed by what had been done to her, she fell into a fit of rage.

Her fury frightened the neighbors, who called the police. When the police arrived, they heard cries and the sound of her throwing things. They entered the house. When they attempted to subdue her, she resisted. So they took her to a mental institution against her will. It took her two days to convince the doctors she wasn't insane. It was especially hard for her to calm down, she said, because her husband did nothing to stop them. Her twin daughters didn't know what to do and were waiting for their dad to come to their mother's defense as she was dragged out of their home kicking and screaming.

The next day I caught the eye of a woman who was attached to an IV pole, standing on the sidewalk in a hospital gown and slippers. She was a walking ghost, a perpetual patient. Her skin hung from her bony frame like loose-fitting clothes. As we approached her, she said matter-of-factly, "I had one of those. When I was 14 years old." Her voice was hoarse from heavy smoking.

"Where did you have the surgery?" Nora had asked her.

"Here. Right here. I wish I hadn't…but too late now, you know? They said I had en-do-me-tri-o-sis!" she said, stressing each syllable of the word sarcastically. "But the pathology came back clean." I lit her next cigarette for her. "Thanks. Wish I could quit, but I'd lose my mind," she said with a laugh. "And I don't have much left to lose." A car pulled up to the curb and the passenger put the window down to take a pamphlet, so I left her alone with Nora.

A few minutes later a young attending physician stood nearby on a smoke break. When I passed him he held out his hand for one of the pamphlets to look at while checking his cell phone messages. A few minutes later he tried to hand the pamphlet back to me, saying, "Thanks, but they don't do unnecessary hysterectomies here."

"Do they do any hysterectomies here?" I asked.

"Of course. If not, why would you be out here?"

"If Brigham and Women's does hysterectomies," I said, "then they do *unnecessary* ones. What's the hysterectomy quota for students in the gynecology rotation?" I asked.

"I don't know," he said, "but they'd never do that to anyone under like 50 years old or something," he said, trying to hand the pamphlet back to me again.

"What does age have to do with it?" I asked. "What age would it be okay for them to take away your sex organs?" He nodded his head, getting my point. "But if you really believe that only women over 50 are hysterectomized here, you should talk with that woman there."

So he did. He and the woman pushing around the IV pole talked for a long time while they smoked. She made several gestures toward the hospital, and he kept shaking his head, looking down at his feet and back at me. Finally, he walked over my way again.

"You know what?" he said as he watched her wheel the IV pole back into the hospital. "You're right. I stand corrected. I don't know what goes on in gynecology, that's not my area, but they totally screwed that woman up. Man, she's got so many problems," he said. "So what is the HERS Foundation?"

He listened intently to my explanation. Nora joined us. At one point I heard him call a friend, saying, "You've got to come out here. There's this protest happening, and this is some scary stuff."

I met Billie Jo Joy of Art & Soul Yoga Studio, my contact for the Boston reading of *un becoming*, through Mitchell Levine, a gynecologist who had spoken at several HERS conferences. The reading featured Paula Plum, who was first-rate in the role of Halley Ridge. And as one audience member said, Jeffrey Korn was "horribly believable" as Dr. Ridge. Mitchell provided insights during the talkback that only a gynecologist could. As we were leaving the studio, one of the actors pulled me aside. We had debated the issues for a long time a few days before the reading, so I was relieved to hear him say, "I learned a lot here today."

The next day at the protest, a guy came out of his house across the street from the hospital, yelling at me, "Get the hell out of here!" I tried to ignore him, but then he screamed, "We live here, and I don't want my kids seeing that!" He crossed the street toward me like he was looking for a fight.

"They're not bad words," I said, "they're medical terms."

"F__ you, I'm calling the police!" he said, as his children looked on.

The police never came.

After the protest Mitchell invited us to spend the rest of the day at the beach with his family. After lounging in the sun a while, Nora and I went for a walk.

We talked about what lay ahead, and at some point Nora said, "We just have a few more things to do before we can change the law."

"How do you see us getting politicians to make this a priority?" I asked.

"There are more than 22 million women alive in this country today whose female organs have been removed from their bodies without informed consent," Nora said. "If only 10% of them changed their vote for President, that would be 2.2 million votes. What would two million votes have meant to Al Gore? What's the value of two million votes to John Kerry or George Bush?" she asked. "And what if 25% of those women voters switched their vote because of this issue? That's five and a half million votes. There are more than 850,000 women HERS has counseled throughout the country, and countless more have avoided hysterectomies when they received information from HERS. What about all the children of hysterectomized women who're angry about what was done to their mothers? It's enough to throw an election—over one issue."

She was right. Changing the laws would require a lot of political finesse, but millions of votes represents a lot of political power. "So, how do you intend to prove that to politicians?" I asked.

"The facts are self-evident," Nora said, "No gynecologist or politician can refute the anatomical facts. Everything we're doing is getting us where we need to go. We will change the law."

EIGHTEEN

Not just a woman's issue.

Cleveland, Ohio—Nora W. Coffey

I realized I was on autopilot when I stepped out of my car at the Philadelphia airport and my bare feet hit the cool parking garage pavement—I'd forgotten my shoes. I was running late, so there was nothing I could do about it. As the US Airways attendants and my fellow passengers tried not to notice, I boarded my flight to Cleveland. When I got to my seat, I phoned back to the office to have my shoes overnighted to the hotel.

The Cleveland Clinic Hospital website says their Center For Specialized Women's Health "provides convenient one-stop shopping for all of a woman's health care needs," including "wellness exams and health care screenings."[58]

Looking for problems in healthy women is unhealthy. It perpetuates the idea that women's bodies are ticking time bombs, ready to explode if they're not routinely inspected for any possible abnormalities. If you scrutinize anyone's body searching for an irregularity, you'll eventually find something "abnormal." This routinized poking and prodding of vaginas, cervixes, uteri, and ovaries is unnatural and causes pain, discomfort, and results in millions of unnecessary procedures and surgeries each year, causing far more damage than they could possibly prevent. The obstetrics and gynecology departments of institutions like the Cleveland Clinic are thought by some to provide the best expertise, but an OB/GYN resident I met when I was a guest speaker at a National

[58] http://my.clevelandclinic.org/womens_health/default.aspx.

Medical Students Association meeting in Crystal City, Virginia, told me hysterectomy was "routine" at Cleveland Clinic.

Two women joined me at the Ohio protest. Valerie was dropped off by her husband Norman, who was on his way to take part in a protest against the Iraq War, a Saturday ritual for him. The other woman had avoided an unwarranted surgery because she received information from HERS.

There was a construction site across the street from our protest. A few of the workers crossed the eight-lane road to get information from us. They tucked the pamphlets into their back pockets before returning to work, avoiding eye contact with us. I spotted one of them reading our pamphlet in his pickup while he ate his lunch, clearly upset by what he was reading.

Although many protestors throughout the year invited me to their homes, I accepted very few invitations. Time alone with my own thoughts had become scarce, and at the end of the protest day I needed a break. But Valerie and I connected immediately, so when she asked me if I'd like to attend a meeting of the Women for Racial and Economic Equality (WREE), I accepted her invitation.

We arrived at a house whose front yard was festooned with large, plastic flamingos and other lawn ornaments. The cyclone fence was also adorned with plastic and rubber insects. Valerie led me around the side of the house to the backyard, which was also a sight to behold—a mosaic of plastic, rubber, and concrete frogs of every color of the rainbow in every nook and cranny.

Soon a few others arrived, and then our host came out of the house. She was gruff, but she was obviously the one in charge.

Each member gave a short report to start off the meeting. I was impressed with the important work its members did for women all over the world. Two of them had recently traveled to Africa.

They worked with heads-of-state at different levels throughout the governments of the countries they visited. They conducted workshops, circulated petitions, and organized demonstrations for female equality.

I drove Valerie home, and along the way she invited me to dinner. Her house was chock full of paintings, drawings, and sculpture. Every possible space was covered with interesting objects and works of art, and each one had a story. Many of them were drawings depicting some kind of violence or terrible ordeal, but all were beautifully done.

Norman said the media showed up to his protest but none had shown up to ours, so Valerie opened the phone book and began making calls. The next day a TV crew showed up, and they all had a good laugh when they saw my bare feet. The local public radio station and the *Cleveland Plain-Dealer* also showed up. That evening my shoes arrived at the hotel at last.

There was a seemingly endless stream of Clevelanders hungry for information about hysterectomy. By then we had distributed many boxes of materials all over the country. Even still, the calls from women desperate for that information remained steady. The following is indicative of the flood of emails HERS receives every day, this one from a woman who was denied that information prior to surgery:

> since the surgery i find myself depressed constantly, i avoid public places, i avoid friends, it took me longer than it should to figure out which direction the wind was blowing from today, I've lost a crucial to my job security badge and have replaced it twice since returning to work....i lost a credit card, my AAA card, my work phone numbers, my DOT card, my

driver's license, i avoided my best friends birthday party...i have to ask myself over and over at work, did i remember to do that...i am losing it. it's over 3 months since the surgery and i at this point wish i wouldn't have survived it. I'm tired all the time, when i get home i can barely walk, so anything i want to do like gardening or rearranging the house, since my daughter left, to put in a hobby area, with table saw and tools I've collected over the years. at work where I'm normally the "take no shit from anyone" type, i find myself meek and all forgiving, very quiet, where i'm normally the one looking to have fun there, i don't stand up for myself anymore... i have no one there to talk to about what's happening to me...they just blow me off with, "more information than i needed to know"...i need a friend, i need information. and I'm broke, what do you need, tax statements? the bills are rolling in and the insurance people are no help other than to say, we don't want her doing anything unnecessary until august, when the doctor gives her a full release... i was out of work for almost three months...even energy assistance gave me a grant. please tell me what to do and how to deal with this...i'm losing my mind!

NINETEEN

Fibroids—hormones, myomectomy, embolization.

Denver, Colorado—Rick Schweikert

Every so often a gynecologist like Ben Thamrong makes the headlines. He's the Manhattan gynecologist who was convicted of Medicaid fraud after being arrested for offering $1,500 and a watch to a state health department investigator. Thamrong was ordered to surrender his license to practice, and was "stricken from the roster of physicians in the State of New York."[59]

The suspended licenses and arrests of gynecologists for bilking the government is the tip of the iceberg of the problem of hysterectomy in this country. The larger offense they commit—removing female organs without informed consent—is legal. Until performing hysterectomies without informed consent is made illegal too, it will continue to go largely unpunished.

Gynecologists become enraged when the facts about hysterectomy are made public. But when the latest medical cash cows and hysterectomy "alternatives" like ablation and embolization are marketed to women, doctors often contradict each other within the same medical journal. In the *American Family Physician*, Steven Janney Smith, a doctor at LaGrange Memorial Hospital in Illinois, writes:

> As an alternative to hysterectomy, uterine fibroid embolization (UFE) avoids the complications and side effects associated with hysterectomy, which include a six-week recovery period, a

---

[59] Barron, James, "Gynecologist Is Arrested On Charges of Bribery," *New York Times*, January 31, 1992.

2 percent risk of postoperative bleeding and a
15 to 38 percent risk of a postoperative febrile
illness. A decrease in sexual function, depression and an increased incidence of cardiovascular disease have also been reported following
hysterectomy.[60]

In the same journal, John Buek of Georgetown University
School of Medicine argues the opposite: "Definitive surgery with
hysterectomy improves most patients' symptoms with minimal effects on sexual function."[61] Finally, *American Family Physician* also
published "ACOG Releases Guidelines on Management of Adnexal
Masses" under the heading "HYSTERECTOMY AND OOPHOREC-
TOMY" which says, "the extent of surgery usually depends on the
diagnosis, patient's age, and the patient's desire for ovarian function or fertility."[62] If a guideline was published under the heading
PENECTOMY AND ORCHIECTOMY, it's unlikely anyone would
say that removal of the penis and testicles depends on a man's age
and his desire to maintain penile and testicular function.

It was always nice when one of the protests happened to
have been scheduled in a town where a friend or family member
lived. The Colorado protest was special to me because it wasn't until I wrote *un becoming* that I discovered that a dear friend in Denver had been hysterectomized many years before. It's a testimony
to the power of what's not said in this country that I can't use her
real name here. I'll call her Anna. Her story, along with that of
another woman I met in Denver named Carla Dionne, is a good

[60] Smith, Steven Janney, "Uterine Fibroid Embolization," *American Family Physician*,
June 15, 2000.
[61] Buek, John, "Management Options for Uterine Fibroid Tumors," *American Family
Physician*," May 15, 2007.
[62] Graham, Lisa, "ACOG Releases Guidelines on Management of Adnexal Masses,"
American Family Physician, May 2008.

example of how what isn't said can sometimes be of greater consequence than what is said.

When I was preparing for the opening of *un becoming* at the 45th Street Theater in New York, a mutual friend of Anna's and mine called to say, "Well you know Anna had one, right?" I began to wonder how many women I knew had been hysterectomized without my knowing about it. It might be in a theater with me, I thought, where they'd make that first crushing realization about why they had so many post-hysterectomy problems.

I decided to broach the subject rather than wait for Anna to do so, but I didn't have to. She called me, and almost without introduction said, "I want to give you my support, and I'll be there for you, but I had a hysterectomy and it was the best thing I ever did."

"Anna, you're married to a great guy and you have kids and grandkids. Surely you don't mean to say that having your female organs removed was the best thing you ever did."

"I had to have it, Rick," she said coolly. "I had fibroids that were pre-cancerous."

I then asked her about her health since the surgery, and the conversation took another familiar turn.

The first of Anna's three suicide attempts came in the first year after her hysterectomy, but she said that was due to depression related to her complicated childhood. She was diagnosed with manic-depression, had back surgery, and began sleeping in a separate bedroom from her husband after she was hysterectomized in a hospital that was part of the massive corporation that employed her.

Anna was the first person to reserve a ticket to see the premiere of *un becoming* in New York. On the way out of the theater everyone received a HERS pamphlet and a notice regarding the upcoming Protest & Play tour. Denver was on the schedule, so Anna and I talked about spending time together when I got into town. But regarding the central message of the play, she said nothing.

Five months later I was in Denver getting the protest underway at Exempla St. Joseph Hospital. St. Joseph's is a popular name for hospitals, including the one where I was born in Omaha. *Exempla*, the Latin plural form of *exemplum*, is a word that means something like "anecdotes that illustrate moral arguments." Their website says, "Most women do not have complications after a hysterectomy." But it's not possible to sever the nerves, blood supply, and ligaments that attach to the uterus and then remove a sex organ that supports the bladder and the bowel without adverse effects.

Anna didn't join us at the protest because, among other reasons, she was employed by the corporation that owned Exempla. The hospital was located in a quiet neighborhood, but we handed out a lot of materials to people walking from the garage to the hospital.

There was a woman walking back and forth on the opposite sidewalk, furiously taking notes while staring at us. I thought maybe she was a journalist. At some point she left, and I didn't think anymore about it, until I met a woman who looked just like her later that afternoon at the El Centro Su Teatro reading of *un becoming*.

Su Teatro was one of two theater companies to respond to our request for proposals to produce readings of *un becoming* in Denver. The role of Susan Herse, a character who is hysterectomized in the play, was played by a woman named Yolanda, who was herself hysterectomized. It was only the second time an actress with first-hand experience with the issues played Susan. Because Su Teatro was short one actor, I played the role of Dr. Ridge.

Anna said little during the talkback, but another woman in the last row was very vocal. Anna observed her closely. The seating at Su Teatro was raked, so the stage lighting was between us and the audience. I blocked my eyes to get a better look at the woman. She had bushy, shoulder-length, sandy-blond hair, and she wore eyeglasses, similar to the person I thought was a journalist at the protest. She talked excitedly in incomplete sentences, and she brought up uterine artery embolization as an alternative treatment to hysterectomy. So we addressed her questions with Nora's standard fibroid "lecture."

Fibroids are benign growths of muscle and connective tissue. They grow until women reach menopause, with a rapid growth spurt generally occurring in the late 30s to early 40s, and another growth spurt just before menopause. At menopause they tend to gradually shrink to a negligible size and calcify.

Fibroids aren't a disease. If you've got them it's because they're part of your genetic blueprint. They rarely cause any problems. But submucosal fibroids—located in the endometrium (the inside layer of the uterus)—can cause heavy menstrual bleeding and pain when large blood clots are passed during menstruation. Sometimes the heavy bleeding can make it difficult for women to manage their daily lives, and in some instances it can cause anemia (abnormally low levels of red blood cells) resulting in iron deficiency.

The best way to increase iron levels is to eat liver. If you don't like liver, you might find it more palatable to eat it the way it's served in Japan—by sautéing or broiling it and then dipping it in soy sauce—or by buying cooked chopped liver and adding soy sauce. Dark leafy green vegetables such as collard greens, kale, or spinach are also high in iron, but they can't restore iron levels as quickly as liver.

Doctors like Anna's often tell women their fibroids might turn into cancer, a condition known as a leiomyosarcoma. But less than 1% of fibroids are cancerous.

Doctors also tell women fibroids will damage their kidneys or bowels by pressing on them, but that too is extremely rare. Women who develop fibroids often don't have any symptoms and don't know they have them unless a doctor tells them.

Both estrogen and progesterone stimulate fibroid growth. Many doctors prescribe progesterone to stop heavy menstrual bleeding and reduce the size of fibroids, but both hormones make them grow.[63] Doctors also recommend "natural" progesterone yam creams that manufacturers claim will shrink fibroids, but they too generally make fibroids grow. Eating certain foods like tofu (or any soy products) can also stimulate abnormally high production of estrogen, especially in women who eat large amounts of it.

Small submucosal fibroids (4cm or less) that cause heavy bleeding can be shelled out in a procedure called a hysteroscopic resection. A hysteroscope is inserted through the vagina, into the cervix, and then into the uterus. A tool is attached to the scope and the surgeon chips away at the fibroid until nothing remains but the shell. Submucosal fibroids that are larger than 4cm can't be removed hysteroscopically. Fibroids larger than 4cm can be removed with myomectomy.

[63] Maruo, Takeshi et al, "Effects of progesterone on uterine leiomyoma growth and apoptosis," *Steroids*, 2000; Rein, Mitchell S. et al, "Progesterone—A critical role in the pathogenesis of uterine myomas," *American Journal of Obstetrics and Gynecology*, 1995.

Myomectomy is the surgical removal of fibroids, leaving the uterus intact. It's still a major operation, but like a hysteroscopic resection it leaves the uterus intact. Any doctor who says a myomectomy can't be performed because of the large size, number, or location of fibroids is simply wrong. Here's what they should say, but rarely do: "I don't have the skill to perform a myomectomy, so I'll recommend you to a more competent surgeon who does."

If you determine that your fibroids should be removed and you find a doctor who claims she or he has the skill to perform a myomectomy, the following questions will be helpful in determining if the doctor has consistently good outcomes with the surgery:

> 1) Are you board certified in gynecology? The desired answer would of course be "yes." Many doctors flunk their gynecology boards multiple times, so it's a minimal expectation that they've passed their boards in their area of expertise.
> 2) How many myomectomies have you performed? It's best to choose a doctor who has performed at least 50.
> 3) How many of the myomectomies you've performed started out as a myomectomy, but ended in a hysterectomy? Answer: More than 2 out of 50 is too many, and you should find a different doctor.
> 4) This is the most important question of all: How many of the women you've performed myomectomies on received a blood transfusion? If the doctor answers you with something like, "It's a really bloody, complicated surgery," then you know you've got the wrong doctor. In that doctor's hands, myomectomy may be a bloody, complicated surgery, but it's generally not for a skilled surgeon. More than 2 blood transfusions in 50 myomectomies is too many.

5) How do you control bleeding during the surgery? You want a doctor who either uses the drug Pitressin or Vasopressin. These drugs are injected directly into the uterus, which causes it to temporarily blanche and diminishes the blood flow. Another acceptable method is a tourniquet, or a combination of a tourniquet and one of these drugs.
6) Finally, if you're told you need to be given the drug Lupron to undergo a myomectomy, then you've got the wrong doctor.

The woman in the back of the audience at Su Teatro was talking about a procedure called uterine artery embolization (UAE). It's been renamed uterine fibroid embolization (UFE), apparently for marketing reasons, because the use of the accurate term "artery embolization" is alarming to women. As Robert Mendelsohn M.D. once said to Nora, gynecologists won't stop performing hysterectomies "until they have another more profitable procedure waiting in the wings." UAE is one such surgery.

It involves essentially starving the fibroids of blood supply by occluding (blocking) the arteries that feed them. A surgeon injects embolic material, such as tiny plastic or gelatin balls, polyvinyl alcohol particles, microspheres, embospheres, gel foam, or even metal coils into the femoral artery, and then into the uterine artery that supplies blood to the fibroid. The idea is that the embolic material will then block the blood supply to the fibroids. Theoretically the fibroids will shrink.

One of the problems is that the fibroids share the same blood supply as other organs, including the uterus, ovaries, and external genitalia. When the blood supply to any part of your body is blocked, the tissue that depends on that blood supply may become necrotic. It can die. The idea of UAE is to only target the fibroids, but if the fibroid tissue does become necrotic it can also cause sepsis (systemic infection), as is noted in numerous articles and studies.[64]

When a doctor obstructs the artery that provides blood flow to the fibroid, he or she might also inadvertently cut off the blood supply to that part of the uterus, and the uterus itself may become necrotic. FDA maintains a database of hundreds of reported complications of UAE. Although it details only a small percentage of the actual number of adverse results (the only complication that must be reported is death), it's a significant number. The Adverse Events database can be accessed by going to "FDA Maude" on the FDA website and entering the search terms "uterine artery embolization" or "uterine fibroid embolization."

There's a long list of adverse effects listed under medical journal references at www.uterinearteryembolization.com, including misembolization (the migration of the embolic material to the legs and other organs, such as the ovaries), sexual dysfunction, and death. HERS has counseled many women with permanent, disabling damage from UAE. Some women experience necrosis of the uterus (leading to a hysterectomy that wasn't necessary before the UAE), necrosis of the vagina, the buttocks, bladder, bowel, and kidney. And many women who call HERS experience a loss of ovarian function, resulting in a de facto castration.

Although UAE does sometimes stop bleeding caused by a fibroid, the relief may be temporary but the embolic material remains in the body for the rest of the woman's life and can cause

---

[64] Martino, Martin A. et al, "Sepsis Leading to Emergent Hysterectomy After Uterine Artery Embolization," *Journal of Gynecologic Surgery*, December 1, 2005; Pelage, J. etal, "Fatal Sepsis after Uterine Artery Embolization with Microspheres," *Journal of Vascular and Interventional Radiology*, April 2004.

other health problems. It can't be removed from the vascular system.

Nor does UAE always shrink fibroids or stop them from continuing to grow. We won't know just how dangerous UAE is until the effects of long-term exposure to radiation (fluoroscopy, allowing doctors to see inside the artery) and the injection of plastic balls and metal coils into the human bloodstream plays itself out in the lives of millions of women. The procedure is being tested in the open market, and women are the human test animals. Recently a 41 year-old woman died two days after a doctor performed a UAE on her.

> I am reporting this for my friend who had this procedure done last week and died as a result of it. The procedure was done at North Ridge Hospital. The procedure was stopped mid way thru as her breathing had become very difficult. The information that we have is that the particles infiltrated her lungs—2 days later her heart stopped. We want it to be known and reported.

HERS works with FDA to post the UAE complications that get reported, but that accounts for only a small percentage of the actual number of bad outcomes. HERS also facilitates the reporting when the hospital, doctor, and/or device manufacturer fail to do so. Although FDA recommends reporting adverse effects, doctors and hospitals aren't required to, except in the event of death. This means that other serious, disabling complications such as chronic severe pain, inability to walk, or outcomes that require fulltime care usually aren't reported. Reporting is recommended, but voluntary. And admitting flaws in treatment isn't good for business.

In this way we answered the woman's questions about UAE in the Su Teatro talkback, but she seemed increasingly frustrated and angry with the facts about UAE and the experiences women report to HERS. Finally, she fell silent. Afterwards I followed her outside to thank her for her comments. When I caught up with her, she asked, "You don't know who I am, do you?"

"No, should I?"

"Well, I'm *Carla Dionne!*" she said.

"You're Carla Dionne of the National Uterine Fibroid Foundation?"

According to their website, NUFF is a "not for profit public benefit corporation organized to engage in charitable, educational and scientific activities related to the care and treatment of women who have uterine fibroids or related conditions of the reproductive system." NUFF provides an online list of its sponsors and donors. The first company on the list of sponsors is Biosphere Medical, a company that manufactures embolic materials (plastic balls) commonly used in UAE, which carries the registered trademark "Embosphere Microspheres." [65]

If you visit cafepress.com/nuff, NUFF offers t-shirts and buttons that say "Ask me about Uterine Fibroid Embolization," hats, sweatshirts, camisoles, bumper stickers, journals, mugs, mouse pads, license plate holders, and even the "Myoma Free Teddy Bear." *Myoma* is another name for *fibroid.* The teddy bear has a t-shirt emblazoned with "Myoma Free with Womb for Ovaries!" There are no "Ask me about Myomectomy" t-shirts and buttons.

Dionne herself underwent a UAE, and here's what she wrote about it in a journal she published online at www.uterinefibroids.com:

---

[65] http://nuff.org/.

- "hot flashes and night sweats"
- "crying in pain" so badly, she says, that she told the nurses to "just kill me and get it over with"
- loss of peripheral and "distance vision"…"the blood vessels that send the eye signal to the brain," she says, "apparently have had 'something' occur to them"
- coughing fits "quickly joined by vomiting and uncontrollable spurts of urination," although later she yells at the doctor for suggesting that she has bladder problems as a result of the UAE
- sexual dysfunction—"This is one area of my UAE that I would have to register in as experiencing a profound loss," she says, "so deeply felt that it can't be expressed in words strong enough without causing tears and an emotional flood of senses."
- Loss of uterine orgasm—"I've now concluded that they are gone forever," she says, in a way that mirrors "women who've experienced sexual dysfunction after a hysterectomy." The problem is, she says, "Doctors aren't telling patients of this potential consequence and I'm none too happy about it."

One of the journal entries dated Monday, November 16, 1998 says that a Dr. Broder asked her, "Did anyone ever discuss myomectomy with you?" Dionne answered yes, two gynecologists suggested it to her, but, "Neither gyn wanted to do the myomectomy." However, when Dionne was interviewed by Paul Indman, he asked, "No one offered you a myomectomy?" and Dionne answered, "No, no one ever offered me a myomectomy." But then when he asked her if she'd had a myomectomy after the UAE, she said yes. Indman then pointed out the obvious: "So now that you've had an embolization and still had to have surgery about that, do you feel that the embolization was a bad thing since you needed surgery?" Dionne replied, "I don't, and I'd choose it again."[66]

Dionne and I talked on the front steps of Su Teatro for a short while. She said she'd send me information about UAE, but I never received it.

Anna, Nora, and I had lunch at the Mercury Café, where the second Denver reading would be staged. Anna picked up one of the HERS pamphlets on the table and began reading it. I was surprised to see it in her hands, because we still hadn't said a word to each other about hysterectomy since our conversation six months earlier. Anna pointed her finger at the long list of adverse effects. As she moved her finger down the list she said, "That one's me… and that one's me…and that one's me." I excused myself, leaving Anna alone with Nora so they could talk.

The next day after the protest Nora and I drove up into the Colorado Rockies west of Denver. We stopped at a cafe with hummingbird feeders on the corners of an outdoor deck, and Nora gave pamphlets to everyone there.

That evening I spent more time with Anna. She talked about how a lot of people are only interested in looking at the sunny side of life, but how that's only half of the picture. The next day I bought a pair of rose-colored sunglasses and wrapped them in a note, telling her sometimes it's okay to only look at the sunny side of life.

---

[66] Indman, Paul, "Paul Indman, MD with Carla Dionne, Executive Director of the National Uterine Fibroid Foundation (NUFF)," *OBGYN.net*, http://www.obgyn.net/hysteroscopy/hysteroscopy.asp?page=/avtranscripts/aagl2001-dionne1, November 2001.

TWENTY

Clear and present danger.

Manchester, New Hampshire—Nora W. Coffey

Three protestors met me at the Manchester Elliott Hospital. Not long into the protest, Darlene informed me that a car had veered toward her, as if trying to hit her. I thought she was joking, but she was sure it was a deliberate attempt to run her over.

A short while later the same driver returned to make another attempt at one of the other protestors. And then it seemed like someone swerved to hit me, so I had to jump out of the way. And then it happened again. And again. I jumped out of the way of one car gunning for me only to run into the side of a slow moving truck. I was knocked to the ground, but I wasn't injured. And the same driver who aimed for Darlene came back at least three more times. There were a few close calls in other cities, but it wasn't just one driver gunning for us in Manchester. We started looking out for each other, but the longer we were out there the more vulnerable we were.

Several hospital representatives stood out front watching us. We alternated between handing pamphlets to people who were eager for the information and running for our lives. Before long a security guard came out to harass us. In an increasingly threatening and menacing tone he said they were calling the police because the hospital insisted that we leave. Several police cars cruised by, glaring at us, but none stopped to question our protest.

I think of New Hampshire as a peaceful, serene, "live free or die" kind of place, but that slogan took on a new meaning for me. In this instance it was more like "live free and you might be run down for it," or, "live free somewhere else or die." Many people yelled obscenities at us, and I was more threatened and at risk in Manchester than anywhere else in the country.

The people who were menacing us, though, were greatly outnumbered by those who were grateful. While most people in cars took materials from us, few people walking by did. In fact, they seemed frightened, as if they were afraid they were being watched. They crossed the street to avoid us or walked around us in a wide berth, too scared to come near. Many women put their passenger side windows down to get information from us only to have the man behind the wheel step on the gas so they couldn't take a pamphlet.

It came to my attention that during the protest Darlene was telling people that HERS is "anti-abortion." I told her that although some of the protestors who joined us had strong opinions on the subject, our protest had nothing to do with abortion, and this wasn't the place to address any issue other than hysterectomy. "But it's what people in Manchester want to hear," she said.

While that may have been true for her and some others, hysterectomy spans all sides of every issue and all political affiliations—the people who support our mandate are Democrats, Independents, Socialists, Republicans, Green Party members, etc.

"While you're out here distributing HERS materials," I said, "you're representing an organization that has made every attempt to be inclusive of all people, regardless of their political or religious stance on any issue. Every woman with a uterus is at risk of being damaged by hysterectomy. HERS doesn't exclude any person or group, because that would be antithetical to our mandate."

Darlene said if she couldn't talk about abortion and express her view that it was every woman's responsibility to procreate, then she wouldn't protest with us. I agreed that if that was the case she shouldn't return the next day.

It was one o'clock and time to quit. Although she was visibly angry, I walked Darlene back to the parking lot. She didn't offer to help carry the protest signs or boxes of materials. As I prepared to leave, she slammed things around the back of her pickup.

Then Darlene did something astonishing. As I packed my trunk, she raced her pickup through the parking lot and veered wildly toward me, like she was trying to run me over. Then she screeched her tires and peeled out of the parking lot. Just minutes before she was talking to me about her Christian faith and doing "God's work," and now here she was trying to run me over. I was stunned.

The next day the security guard came out to harass me again. When I didn't leave he swore at me, and then he spat on me. We can only imagine what Manchester Elliot Hospital does to women inside those walls if that's an acceptable way of treating people outside on public property.

I don't frighten easily. It's one of the consequences of hysterectomy and castration. As Halley says in Rick's play, the worst thing that could've been done to me has already been done. Halley says, "Only I have to know that's true." But trying to get information out to women in this city put us in serious danger. And perhaps more than anywhere else, I felt like women who enter Manchester Elliott Hospital might be in grave potential danger.

No wonder so many of the women I met there were sad, lonely, and angry. Rapid City wins the award for the friendliest and most welcoming city. Manchester wins the award for being the most hostile and unwelcoming.

TWENTY-ONE

Help with weight, insomnia, memory loss…

Portland, Maine—Nora W. Coffey

One of our fellow protestors in Maine, a woman named Mary, said she was "badgered" into hysterectomy without informed consent by her gynecologist, Christiane Northrup.

Northrup is one of gynecology's leading celebrities. In a book she wrote, and in her numerous television and radio interviews, Northrup says hysterectomy should only be performed as a last result. But Mary tells a different story.

On her website titled "A Question of Accountability (my ordeal as a patient of Dr. Christiane Northrup MD)," Mary says:

> [Northrup] said, "That's it, that's it, you're having a hysterectomy first thing tomorrow morning! I'm going to do as I was taught (i.e. in medical school). This time I'm taking charge!" She told me that she would no longer be my doctor if I refused to submit to the surgery. Although I was given four units of blood (which for me added fear to the trauma), I was not given anything to stop the bleeding. Under these conditions I saw no way out and I was too exhausted and vulnerable to fight back, so, under duress, I signed the release. Yet even then, I was still literally begging Christiane to leave my uterus in and remove only the fibroid tumors. (the medical records note that I was "reluctant to go to surgery") I recall her saying, "Well, you know you've tried *everything*." Everything?!?[67]

---

[67] Cupp, Mary L., "A Question of Accountability (my ordeal as a patient of Dr. Christiane Northrup MD)," http://users.rcn.com/cabbidge/Index.html.

Mary was late arriving at the protest, and I was already set up at the Maine Medical Center when I spotted her. Driving wasn't easy for her anymore, let alone walking and standing on the street with a sign distributing materials for two hours. Her struggles were obvious, watching her climb the hill to meet me, but as she said, "I wouldn't have missed this for the world."

We spent most of our time talking about how she believed she was duped by Northrup, about her numerous problems since the surgery, and about the immense anger she felt knowing these problems would never go away.

There was a lot of foot traffic, and we set up our protest beside one of the walls of a parking garage where hospital employees took their breaks. Many visitors and hospital staff came out to speak with us.

One employee crossed the street toward us with an unlit cigarette. Every step seemed painful, and she seemed oblivious to the traffic bearing down on her. When the light changed faster than she could cross the street, the cars had no choice but to wait impatiently for her to reach the curb. As she approached me I handed her one of the pamphlets. She took it, but said, "Yeah? Well, it saved my life!" She walked around the corner and lit her cigarette.

"Why did you have the surgery?" I asked.

"Because I was bleeding like a stuck pig, that's why!"

A few other women sat on a wall nearby. One of them launched into a tirade about how she too had heavy bleeding and would've died without the surgery.

"If you had heavy menstrual bleeding and were passing large blood clots, you most likely had submucosal fibroids, which are benign growths in the lining of your uterus," I said. "But no one ever needs a hysterectomy for fibroids."

The first woman, who'd gone around the corner to smoke, returned to the hospital. Her voice cracking, she said, "You folks don't know what you're talking about."

The next day one of the women returned and casually took a pamphlet. "I didn't know there was any other choice," she said. She looked at the pamphlet for a while and then nonchalantly began telling me about all the problems she was having. She remained there for the rest of the protest talking with me about how sick she was since the surgery.

Some people think when it comes to questions of health, hospital employees have an advantage because of where they work. In many ways, the exact opposite is true. The closer women are to a hospital, and the better their medical coverage is, the more vulnerable they are.

One of the reasons women don't talk about the way they feel after the surgery is they know this would sound crazy and bizarre to anyone who hasn't experienced it. The changes in your outward appearance aren't so obvious to strangers who don't see your hair falling into the sink each morning and your skin drying to the point of burning— most of the damage is unseen. Although they may sense something has changed, they can't see the sadness and melancholy of knowing you'll never be the same again. Your family and friends may try to understand, but it's too terrifying for most people to allow themselves to truly comprehend the inhumanity of what's being done to women. It's often too painful for family and friends to accept the horror of a loved one's irreparable pain and suffering.

One of the things that struck me in Maine (and elsewhere too, but particularly there) was the number of hysterectomized women who become thorough researchers of all alleged miracle cures to their post-operative problems. They ask if I've heard about this or that chemical or vitamin or diet or drug. I think I've heard them all, until some doctor dreams up another alleged cure to give women back their sex life, their energy, and their lust for life. After spending a small fortune on these magic bullet cures, it doesn't take long to discover they don't deliver what they promise—none of them can restore the functions of the female organs.

The women who call HERS seek the right combination of synthetic hormones, they switch doctors, they consider suicide, they pray to a higher power, they change relationships, and they switch doctors again. They ask if there's a "natural" product their doctors don't know about, because no doctor seems to be able to provide them with relief. But there's no remedy, no cure, no miracle concoction from the rain forest, no organic substance from the garden, and certainly nothing for them in any pharmacy or doctor's office that can undo the damage. And it's understandable to hold out hope that things will improve, no matter how impossible that may be.

It's a testimony to the human spirit that so many women are able to live with all these problems. They join the protest without knowing that I too cope with constant physical pain and profound fatigue. What I do is by dint of inordinate struggle—it's not because of any cure. The only cure is to make hysterectomy without informed consent illegal. Many people refuse to accept it by denying it. We—and women like Mary—refuse to accept it by working to change the law.

On my last night in Maine I found an excellent restaurant called Fore. I sat near a table with three women, and I couldn't help but overhear their conversation. At some point they began talking about hysterectomy. One of them was scheduled for surgery. At the end of the day, I needed a break, but in a country where another woman is hysterectomized every minute, the odds of sitting next to a woman who's confronted with hysterectomy are pretty good.

Although I welcome any opportunity to inform the public, I wasn't in the mood to engage them and was there in search of a quiet oasis. But at some point I couldn't tolerate the party-like atmosphere surrounding what was about to be done to her. So I took three pamphlets from my bag and gave one to each of them. They looked up as if I'd just landed from outer space. I returned to my table without a word.

Two of them (one of them being the woman who was scheduled for surgery) began reading the pamphlets, while the other made an effort to revive the conversation where they'd left off. But the party atmosphere had vanished. So I vanished too, into my solitude, enjoying the meal and catching up on some reading.

When I left, the one scheduled for surgery turned around, saying, "Hey," stopping me. I cringed, because I wasn't in the frame of mind to put up with cynical comments or for her to hand the pamphlet back to me because her doctor had already made her mind up for her. But after a pause she said, "Thank you. I appreciate this."

'One at a time,' I thought. It's how women are damaged, and it's how women avoid being damaged. One at a time.

Another protest was done, but the information we left behind would have a ripple effect as it was passed from woman to
woman. Next week we'd be moving from one corner of America to
the other, one protest closer to ending this conspiracy of silence.

TWENTY-TWO

Endometrial ablation and hyperplasia.

Anchorage, Alaska—Rick Schweikert

Providence Alaska Medical Center was another hospital where there were no public sidewalks to speak of. We tucked pamphlets under windshield wipers, handed them out to students, and hit the coffee shops, bookstores, and libraries. And there were a lot of them—judging by Nora's tried-and-true method for determining a city's livability index by the number of coffee shops and bookstores it has per capita, Anchorage is a very livable city.

There were only two performances of *un becoming* that Nora and I didn't attend, and both were in Homer, Alaska. Both Pier One Theater in Homer and Cyrano's Theatre Company in Anchorage responded to our request for proposals, so once again we accepted both. We looked into taking a puddle-jumper plane down to attend the Pier One readings, but we couldn't make it work. HERS received a surprising number of calls from people who attended the Homer readings, including one from a friend of a woman who met her future husband at the reading.

I had never worked with a group of actors who seemed to know each other better than the actors at Cyrano's, and their reading was superb too. The general response from the audience was not to question the central issue of the play, but more to question the need for the play in the first place. As one of the actors said, "I just can't imagine women up here letting any doctor operate on them unless she had to crawl on her hands and knees to the hospital already half dead."

After each reading and interview we usually got a thank-you note or two and an email from a woman who was told she needed surgery but realized she didn't. But before we even left Anchorage Nora got a call from a woman named Sandy who heard the interview of us on KSKA 91.1.

The first person to call was Sandy's attorney, gathering information for a malpractice case. Not long after Nora hung up with him, Sandy called from the hospital. She was in such bad shape she was waiting to be airlifted to a larger hospital outside Alaska, following a hysterectomy to treat endometriosis. Once she was stabilized and sent home, her lover of ten years left her, she filed for disability because she was in constant pain, and the attorney ultimately declined her case because she signed a consent form.

We also got a call from a doctor who heard the radio interview. Nora said he came across as supportive of our work, telling her, "I pursue non-damaging alternatives to hysterectomy at all costs. And if I ever do a hysterectomy, I do it laparoscopically."

"So you believe that women aren't damaged if you perform hysterectomies laparoscopically?"

"Well," he said, "if I leave the cervix intact, yes."

Nora replied, "So, because it involves morcellating the uterus into small pieces and pulling them out through the navel, you think that because you use a laparoscope she isn't damaged?" After a pause, Nora continued. "If you remove a woman's uterus through her nostrils, it's just as damaging. She'll still lose all of the functions of the uterus, she'll still have nerve damage, she'll still have back problems, she'll never have a uterine orgasm again, she'll lose support to her bladder and bowel, and if the ovaries are removed or cease to function she'll still be castrated. You'll only have succeeded in removing her uterus through her nose instead of her vagina."

"Well, anyway, I try to avoid hysterectomy at all costs," the doctor said, "and before I resort to hysterectomy for heavy bleeding I first try ablation."

Ablation involves burning the endometrium (the inside lining of the uterus) and permanently scarring it. The idea is to scar the endometrium so it can't proliferate. If it can't build-up, there'll be nothing to shed as it naturally does during menstruation. The problem is, even though the endometrium is permanently scarred, the uterus still tries to perform its natural functions. The natural engorgement of blood still occurs, but the lining of the uterus can't build up after it's been burned. Because it can't build up, there's nothing to shed, so the uterus remains engorged with nowhere for the blood to go. That may initially only cause a feeling of fullness in the pelvis, but after a few months of this abnormally induced amenorrhea (suppression of menstruation), many women experience constant, debilitating pain.

In addition to the common occurrence of severe, ongoing pain, the risks of ablation include: possible perforation of the uterus, bowel, or bladder, infection, hemorrhage, thermal injuries to the uterus and other organs, fluid overload, and death.

A doctor begins an ablation by filling the woman's body with fluid intravenously. The amount of fluid must be closely monitored, and every woman is unique in terms of how much her body will tolerate. The surgeon then applies the heat to the endometrium, which causes some of the fluid to evaporate. Some of the fluid is also absorbed into the woman's body, but the amount of evaporation and absorption can't be measured precisely, and women have died from fluid overload of the heart and lungs.

The first method of ablation doctors used to burn and scar the endometrium was electrocautery. Later, rollerball ablation was developed, which involves heating a metal ball sufficiently to burn the endometrium. Rollerball was then replaced with cryo-ablation, which involves burning by freezing. And when cryoablation was finally recognized as just as damaging as all of the other methods, balloon ablation was invented, which involves filling a balloon with an extremely hot substance and inserting it into the uterus. The idea is that a heated balloon will burn the endometrial tissue more slowly, and thus be safer. And after balloon ablation came microwave ablation. But if a doctor said to a man that he was going to scar the inside of his genitals by burning them, it wouldn't make any difference what method was used. It would still damage his sex organs. It makes no difference if it's done slowly or quickly, by heating or freezing or microwave—it's still damaging.

Furthermore, there's no remedy for the problems caused by ablation, because you can't unscar the uterus. The symptoms often worsen with each menstrual cycle because of the unreleased engorgement of menstrual blood, so by the end of the first or second year following ablation, a lot of women are told that hysterectomy is the only option to get relief from the problems caused by it.

Balloon endometrial ablation was invented by Robert S. Neuwirth, who is affiliated with St. Luke's-Roosevelt Hospital at Columbia University in New York. His bio says he introduced techniques "to avoid hysterectomy."[68] But FDA's Manufacturer And User Facility Device Experience Database (MAUDE) reveals that the end result of balloon ablation may be hysterectomy. In those

---

[68] Continuum Health Partners, http://www.docnet.org/physicians/phys_bios.aspx? phys_id=1301.

instances, not only do the balloons and the ablators fail "to avoid hysterectomy," they actually lead to hysterectomy. More specifically, the following is from an article titled "Complications Associated With Global Endometrial Ablation: The Utility of the MAUDE Database":

> RESULTS: …A search of the US Food and Drug Administration MAUDE database yielded reports of 85 complications in 62 patients. These included major complications: eight cases of thermal bowel injury, 30 cases of uterine perforation, 12 cases in which emergent laparotomy was required, and three intensive care unit admissions. One patient developed necrotizing fasciitis and eventually underwent vulvectomy, ureterocutaneous ostomy, and bilateral below-the-knee amputations. One of the patients with thermal injury to the bowel died.
> CONCLUSION: Use of the US Food and Drug Administration MAUDE database is helpful in identifying serious complications associated with global endometrial ablation not yet reported in the medical literature.[69]

It's ironic that FDA provides MAUDE—a very helpful forum for the public to see just how damaging these devices and techniques are—while it's responsible for approval of these damaging devices and techniques in the first place. Unfortunately, the way we find out just how dangerous these medical practices are comes only after FDA approves them and millions of people are injured. Only after deaths and public outcry is something finally done. FDA has become an arm of industry and no longer puts public safety first.

---

[69] Gurtcheff, Shawn E. and Sharp, Howard T., "Complications Associated With Global Endometrial Ablation: The Utility of the MAUDE Database," *Obstetrics & Gynecology*, July 2003.

One of the many examples of the interdependent relationship between FDA and the medical industry is what's known as
"preemption." Preemption is a legal doctrine that aims to protect
the medical industry from product liability lawsuits when the device or drug has been approved by FDA. A *New York Times* editorial
explains the perverse problems with this situation:

> The pharmaceutical industry...[is] working
> hard to prevent consumers from filing damage
> suits for injuries caused by federally approved
> drug products... If this perverse legal doctrine,
> known as federal pre-emption, continues to
> spread, the public will be deprived of a vital tool
> for policing companies and unearthing docu-
> ments that reveal their machinations.[70]

Another *Times* article by Gardiner Harris and Alex Berenson, paints an even grimmer picture of FDA oversight:

> A series of independent assessments have
> concluded that the agency is poorly organized,
> scientifically deficient and short of money. In
> February, its commissioner, Andrew C. von
> Eschenbach, acknowledged that the agency fac-
> es a crisis and may not be "adequate to regulate
> the food and drugs of the 21st century." The
> F.D.A. does not test experimental medicines
> but relies on drug makers to report the results
> of their own tests completely and honestly. Even
> when companies fail to follow agency rules,
> officials rarely seek to penalize them.[71]

It's sometimes difficult to discern accurate information
from misinformation...or reliable sources from self-promotion.
The website OBGYN.net, for example, may seem like an informa-

---

[70] Editorial, "The Dangers in Pre-emption," *New York Times*, April 14, 2008.
[71] Harris, Gardiner and Berenson, Alex, "Drug Makers Near Old Goal: A Legal
Shield," *New York Times*, April 6, 2008.

tive site. It lists a Herbert Goldfarb as Editorial Advisor for hysterectomy alternatives and infertility.[72] It also publishes an essay from Goldfarb, where he tells us that the first endometrial ablation was performed in 1981 by "Goldrath and colleagues." Here's a quote from that page:

> ...A study by Unger and Meeks indicated that as many as 34% of women required a hysterectomy within 5 years of ablation, a number that increased with time. A recent report by Martyn and Allan on long-term follow-up of 301 patients having endometrial ablation revealed that after 5 years 27% had required further surgery because of bleeding, and 38% because of pain... Those authors also noted that because the uterine cavity may be scarred by the procedure and no longer patent with the vagina, any subsequent menstrual flow may be forced into the fallopian tubes, causing pain and endometriosis.[73]

Goldfarb is the author of *The No Hysterectomy Option,* a book that tells women they almost never need a hysterectomy. As he says, no matter how you perform an ablation, scarring, menstrual problems, and subsequent surgeries are very common. Goldfarb is also a member of The One-Kilo Club, whose mission is spelled out on their website, onekiloclub.org:

> The ONE-KILO CLUB is an association of pelvic surgeons who are committed to furthering the technical horizons of minimally invasive surgery and who have demonstrated that commitment by their accomplishments. Hence our motto,

[72] http://www.obgyn.net/meet.asp?page=/all_advisors/H_Goldfarb.
[73] Goldfarb, Herbert, "Does Combining Myoma Coagulation with Endometrial Ablation Reduce Subsequent Surgery?" OBGYN.net, http://www.obgyn.net/hysterectomy-alternatives/hysterectomy-alternatives.asp?page=/ah/articles/goldfarb_myoma.

> EX UNGUE LEONEM (By its claw one tells the lion.) The extirpation of a uterus that weighs one kilogram or more without a laparotomy has been chosen as the test of that commitment…

To "extirpate" is to cut out, kill, destroy. The One-Kilo Club, then, is an association of surgeons who believe that cutting out a person's sex organs with a laparoscope is "minimally invasive," but minimally invasive compared to what? There's a poem on their website called "The One-Kilo Lion." One of the lines of that poem says of the uterus, "Please, weigh it accurately, it might be a kilo, as good as gold and diamonds."

ExAblate is yet another device currently being tested on women in American hospitals with FDA's blessing. Like ablation, it brings gold and diamonds to gynecologists, but a lifetime of grief for the women who are damaged by it. It involves burning the fibroid itself, not the entire endometrium. But it's been shown to burn other tissue as well, causing pain and injury that can radiate throughout the pelvis, buttocks, and lower extremities. A report on FDA's MAUDE makes the point very clearly:

> Treatment was stopped when the pt [patient] complained of pain radiating to the left leg and catheter tip. In recovery the lady complained of a sensation of numbness in the left buttock. On closer exam she was found to have decreased sensation throughout the peri-anal and perine-al region as well as the posterior left thigh. She had leaked some faecal matter….

ExAblate involves using high intensity focused ultrasound (HIFU) waves to burn fibroids. HERS recently received an email from a woman who said she underwent ExAblate, but the bleeding returned. She's searching for a doctor who has the skill to perform a myomectomy, but none of the doctors in her area will do it. The reason they're reluctant is that ExAblate creates adhesions that are thicker and larger than the kind of scar made by cutting, so the ExAblate treatment may have made it more difficult, if not impossible, to now perform a myomectomy.

Doctors like the one who called Nora continue to use these devices on unsuspecting women who are led to believe that because it's not a hysterectomy they'll be improved by the newest, most promising ablation to date, using the latest state-of-the-art technology available to perform endometrial destruction.

Probably the most high-profile case of ablation is the one that killed Lisa Smart in 1998. The equipment used to monitor the fluid infiltration during the ablation was operated by a salesman from Johnson & Johnson, the equipment's manufacturer. A *New York Times* article relates the grief suffered by Smart's husband:

> Staring blankly at reporters yesterday, Mr. Smart, a New York City police officer, read from a small sheet of paper: "I am here today because our families have vowed to make sure Lisa did not die in vain. Lisa died because Beth Israel, its doctors and Johnson & Johnson put business ahead of health, ego ahead of common sense and, in the height of arrogance, tried to put their own reputation ahead of the truth."[74]

Most stories of botched surgeries don't make the news headlines. And most women have no idea which gynecologists may have been negligent in the past or which ones had their hospital privileges or licenses to practice suspended. As Nora says, "We can easily find the hits, runs, and errors on any baseball player by picking up a newspaper, but we can't get the runs, hits, and errors on doctors who have our lives in their hands."

[74] Steinhauer, Jennifer, "Hospital Accused of Hiding Details of Woman's Death," *New York Times,* November 10, 1998.

Susan Gilbert of the *New York Times*, also reporting on the tragedy of Lisa Smart's death, draws an apt comparison:

> In the early 1990's seven patients in New York died and 151 were injured during gall bladder surgery because their doctors were inadequately trained in using a laparoscope. One doctor had received no formal instruction; others one- or two-day seminars.[75]

The reason Lisa Smart's case got so much exposure in the *Times* and elsewhere was that she was a young newlywed, her husband was a police officer, and the operator of the equipment was a salesman. How many women die that we don't hear about because it was a "trained surgeon" who killed an older woman?

Ablation is often performed for heavy or continuous bleeding. That kind of bleeding is sometimes caused by endometrial hyperplasia, an abnormal build-up of the endometrium. Hyperplasia progresses slowly through the early, simple, cystic, and then on up the ladder to complex adenomatous hyperplasia with atypia, before becoming a frank endometrial cancer. The two most common factors that can speed up that timeline are hormones and weight. Excess estrogens are stored in fatty tissue. Excess androgens are converted to estrogens in the fatty tissue and stored, which accelerates the hyperplasia's growth.

The first step in determining if you have hyperplasia is a pelvic and transvaginal ultrasound, which evaluates the thickness of the endometrium. The endometrium is thickest before menstruation and thinnest after, so ultrasound should be performed within a day or two after menstruation stops—when the thickness

---

[75] Gilbert, Susan, "Ideas & Trends: No Deus Ex Machina; First Read The Directions, Then Do No Harm," *New York Times*, November 22, 1998.

of the endometrium should be between about 4mm and 7mm. It's common for low-level hyperplasia to develop in perimenopausal women (the beginning of menopause), but it usually spontaneously reverts to normal after menopause.

Most doctors want to first perform an endometrial biopsy (the removal of a small sample of endometrial tissue with a thin, glass, straw-like pipelle), an extremely painful procedure that is inadequate to evaluate the endometrium. It only tells you what's going on in the spot where the tiny endometrial sample was removed.

If an ultrasound reveals that the endometrium is abnormally thickened, it should be confirmed the following month with a repeat ultrasound that's performed not more than a week after menstruation ends to make sure the first one was accurate. If the endometrium remains thickened or if bleeding continues after menstruation for two months in a row, then a D&C (dilation of the cervix and scraping of the lining of the uterus) will both diagnose hyperplasia (it allows a pathologist to determine if it exists, and if so what level) and treat it (because the build up of endometrial tissue is removed during the D&C). Whether or not further treatment is advisable will be determined by the level of hyperplasia.

Although ablation is contraindicated for endometrial hyperplasia, it's commonly performed to stop the heavy bleeding associated with it. Ablation isn't advisable for hyperplasia because it makes it impossible to monitor the endometrium and may mask hyperplasia. The thickness of the endometrium can be monitored with pelvic and transvaginal ultrasound. But after ablation, the lining is scarred and doesn't proliferate as it normally would, so the endometrium can't then be evaluated to see if it's reverting to normal or if the hyperplasia is progressing. So if the hyperplasia continues to progress because it's not being treated, it can invade the myometrium (the middle layer of the body of the uterus). What starts out as a low-level, treatable hyperplasia may develop to a higher level. And if not treated appropriately, it may progress to cancer.

Many women continue to have bleeding after ablation because some areas of the endometrium may have been burned unevenly, inadvertently leaving some of the endometrium to grow. But because of the scarring there's no way of knowing if the bleeding is caused by the ablation or by continuing hyperplasia. At that point women are likely to be told they need a hysterectomy. The women who contact HERS say they would not have consented to ablation in the first place if they had been told about the risks and the appropriate conservative treatment for hyperplasia.

The Spring 2004 edition of *New Growth Opportunities in Medical Technology* is telling:

> The primary motivation behind this report is… a breakout in the growth of the UroGynecology market… While the current market sizes remain fairly modest, investor awareness of these expanding market opportunities is expanding, boosted by items such as American Medical's eye-opening announcement of 80% growth in its women's health business in the fourth quarter of 2003.[76]

One of the subtopics under "TREATMENTS FOR ABNORMAL UTERINE BLEEDING (AUB)" is "Surgery…Hysterectomy

[76] Simpson, Gregory J. and Kouchoukos, Thomas, "Women's Health/Uro Gynecology—Overview & Investment Thesis," *New Growth Opportunities in Medical Technology*, "Focus on Women's Health," Spring 2004.

Remains the Gold Standard." It's the gold standard, all right, and the goldmine. But gynecologists first expand their markets by selling women a D&C, an ablation, and maybe a UAE too before they remove the female organs. It's like leaving money on the table to not perform other treatments before turning to the "gold standard" of unnecessary and damaging surgeries—hysterectomy.

TWENTY-THREE

"I thought I had nothing more to lose."

Providence, Rhode Island—Nora W. Coffey

At only 21 years old, Debbie was told she had endometriosis and was hysterectomized. The surgery damaged her kidney, but the doctor told her "that's normal." In fact, the tissue was dying. At 24 one of her eyes was removed because of a misdiagnosis of glaucoma. At 27 she was also castrated for endometriosis. Six months after her ovaries were removed she developed such severe, chronic pain in her back that her doctor implanted a transcutaneous stimulator (TENS unit) with a remote control to send electrical signals to deaden the pain. Debbie ultimately sued her doctor, and they settled out of court.

The Providence Women & Infant's Hospital website publishes a "Health Encyclopedia" with a "search" option. By searching for "endometriosis" and then clicking on "Surgical Procedures For Endometriosis," they tell us that hysterectomy "is generally considered the most effective treatment for severe endometriosis." As we said in the Indiana chapter, we couldn't disagree more. Debbie herself felt strongly enough to the contrary that she was willing to stand on the street with a sign protesting against it.

Even the Women & Infant's Hospital seems to refute itself on its website by saying, "About 50% of women treated with hysterectomy alone later need another operation due to continued problems with endometriosis." [77] In other words, according to the authors of their website, the odds of hysterectomy solving the

---

[77] http://www.womenandinfants.org/body.cfm?id=388&chunkiid=19393.

problems caused by endometriosis without another operation is about the same odds as flipping a coin. Do they really think that 50/50 odds amount to the "most effective treatment?" What they don't mention is that the odds of experiencing some or all of the adverse effects of hysterectomy are 100%. As mystery writer Ben Hecht said, "Despite all our toil and progress, the art of medicine still falls somewhere between trout casting and spook writing."[78]

Although she was hysterectomized, castrated, had a kidney removed, was legally blind, and in constant pain, Debbie's problems didn't stop her from walking out into the street handing pamphlets through open car windows. Her hearing was extremely sharp, which helped her compensate for her visual impairment, and she was cautious, but it was scary watching her step on and off the curb of that busy street to hand out as much information as other protestors did with 20/20 vision. She said she wouldn't let the doctors take away her ability to help other women.

Her husband sat at a respectful distance across the street watching her. The only available parking was up a steep hill, so he ferried materials back and forth to us.

Early on a nurse came out of the hospital and took a pamphlet from Debbie. As the nurse read the pamphlet, her shoulders drooped. She returned inside the hospital without a word. After that silent encounter Debbie seemed more eager to engage with the public.

After the protest, Debbie was in such pain it would've been difficult for her to walk up the hill to their car. I walked with her husband to the parking lot as she waited. He was mild-mannered and showed no hint of anger in front of Debbie. But when we were

---

[78] Ben Hecht, "Miracle of the Fifteen Murderers," *Colliers*, January 16, 1943.

alone he said Debbie had settled out of court with her doctor because she couldn't stand to be subjected to the requisite physical examinations, as Rhode Island law requires. He was angry about the motives of the medical industry and the carelessness and brutality of the way his wife was treated.

The Providence Women & Infants Hospital website asks:

> What makes you happy, what makes you feel accomplished, what brings you comfort or support, what brings you a sense of peace and wellness? What are your causes? What are your secret indulgences? … E-mail us to let us know. And we'll work to bring you programs, make connections, and leverage our collective strengths to help give you what you want. Imagine the possibilities…[79]

Reading this I wonder, exactly what is the role of our nation's hospitals? To help us imagine our dreams? Women in Rhode Island don't need Providence Women & Infants Hospital to imagine their "secret indulgences." Hospitals perform a service. They make money selling surgeries, procedures, and drugs.

Debbie's daughter joined us for lunch after the protest. She was studying to become a nurse. Just as children who want to fix their dysfunctional families often become psychiatrists, many daughters of damaged women want to learn how to repair and recover the mother they lost to the surgery. But the damage can't be undone.

---

[79] http://www.womenandinfants.org/body.cfm?id=561.

TWENTY-FOUR

Her doctor wouldn't take no for an answer.

Detroit, Michigan—Rick Schweikert

The website for St. Joseph's Hospital in Pontiac, Michigan says this about its new corporate arrangement:

> The Sisters of Mercy Regional Community of Detroit and the Congregation of the Sisters of the Holy Cross have now consolidated their health ministries—Mercy Health Services and Holy Cross Health System—to form a new system. Called Trinity Health, this new system will be sponsored by Catholic Health Ministries. The spirit of this new organization arises from the healing ministry of the Church. The creation of Trinity Health affirms the belief that Catholic health care has a vital future in this country.[80]

The new "system" created by this merger is named after the Christian trinity—God The Father, God The Son, and God The Holy Ghost.

Early on during our protest, a St. Joseph Mercy Oakland Hospital administrator came out to speak with us. Casually dressed, she didn't fit the middle-aged-man-in-a-suit-and-tie stereotype of a hospital administrator.

"This is a Catholic hospital," she said sincerely, "we don't do hysterectomies here."

"Really. Well, this is our 22nd protest of the year," I said, "and many of the women we've spoken with were hysterectomized in

---

[80] http://www.stjoesoakland.org/aboutus_history.htm.

Catholic hospitals. Like that woman over there," I said, pointing toward Sue.

The Detroit protest fell on Sue's wedding anniversary. She and her husband Brian had planned to spend it in Paris but changed their plans when they heard about the protest. When they walked up, Brian asked, "Is there a problem?" I told them what the hospital administrator said. In a calm and diplomatic tone, Brian explained how a female gynecologist at a Catholic hospital bullied Sue into a hysterectomy over a period of years.

Sue then described the gynecologist pacing in circles around her telling her she was being irresponsible, as Sue sat on the examination table half naked. The doctor said she wouldn't take no for an answer, that the hysterectomy had to be done right away. Finally Sue gave in—she was hysterectomized in a hospital that's now part of Trinity Health. The surgery was unwarranted, and the surgeon was a woman who was later made head of the department.

"After the surgery Sue could barely move," Brian told the administrator. "She sat on my lap crying for weeks and weeks. And believe me, that's not like her. Sue was a strong woman who ran a Christmas tree farm, raised a family, and was an artist to boot. There was nothing she couldn't do. But after the surgery there was nothing I could do but hold her. She'd get into the car and drive down roads she knew like the back of her hand, but she'd get lost. Her balance was off, she was in pain, and she was just confused so much of the time."

"Today's our anniversary," Sue said. "We have a strong relationship, and we used to have a wonderful sex life, but now all that's gone. I'm just so lucky to have a wonderful guy to stick with me. That's how we found HERS, and you should feel lucky we're out here in front of your hospital helping women."

Sue and Brian have now spoken at HERS conferences and have joined Nora and me at speaking engagements, Women's Studies conferences, and media interviews, like the one titled "Sexless After Surgery?" conducted by 20/20, where they were interviewed on their Christmas tree farm in Michigan.[81]

Sue and Brian weren't exactly protesting types. As is the case with most first-timers, they were a bit awkward out of the gate. They were protesting on a public street, after all, where they might be seen by friends and family. But they were effective protestors. Brian would cock his head in a way that seemed to say, "Now listen here, you! This is good information, and I advise you to take a look at it," as he thrust the pamphlet with an outstretched hand. It was rare for someone to say no to them.

Probably the most prolific protestor of the year was a woman named Joan who also lived in the Detroit area. Joan was willing to talk about hysterectomy with anyone and everyone, from the airline agent to the hotel concierge. Because of her we had a very accommodating venue for the reading of *un becoming* in Detroit, which she single-handedly publicized and got ample media coverage for.

Joan was hysterectomized when she was diagnosed with an early stage of endometrial cancer. Along with her uterus, the doctor unnecessarily removed her ovaries and pelvic lymph nodes. We know that the removal of the lymph nodes was unnecessary, because if the cancer had spread to them no amount of surgery

[81] "Sexless After Surgery? Women, Doctors Say Hysterectomies May Be Detrimental to Sexual Health," *20/20*, ABC News, August 22, 2002.

would've saved her life. And if the cancer had been localized, then there would've been no reason to take out her lymph nodes. Not only did the doctor and nurses neglect to inform her of the aftermath of hysterectomy prior to the surgery, they neglected to inform her that, as a result of the lymphadenectomy, she'd be at high risk for lymphedema, high fluid retention caused by problems with the lymph nodes.

Lymphedema occurs when lymphatic circulation is altered. Lymph fluid accumulates in the extremities and abdomen, causing severe swelling and the sensation of "pins and needles," if not a total loss of motion in those areas. No one mentioned she'd have to spend a couple hours wrapping her legs in the morning before starting each day and before going to bed each night. Nor did they tell her that whenever she went anywhere for any length of time she'd have to bring three pairs of shoes, because her feet swelled throughout the day and her shoe size increased every few hours.

Beyond these substantial inconveniences, lymphedema can be a dangerous condition. Cellulitis—an acute inflammation of the connective tissue of the skin—can develop and spread to the lungs and brain. It's fatal if not contained. At dinner or while riding in the car, profound fatigue (a symptom of cellulitis) would sometimes catch up with Joan, and she'd unexpectedly fall asleep. She also had severe gastro-intestinal problems stemming from the radiation she received as a follow-up to the surgery.

At the Detroit protest Joan sat on a lawn chair under a tree in the center island of the boulevard. Every fifteen minutes or so she had to elevate her swollen leg. In spite of the increased difficulties, it seemed like every time I looked up someone was honking their horn at her, giving her the thumbs-up, and sometimes screeching to a halt so she could hand a pamphlet to them through their car window. For the most part Detroit was receptive to our message.

Joan kept a diary of her HERS protest experiences, which included Detroit, Chicago, New York, Minneapolis, Philadelphia, Dallas, Atlanta, and Washington DC. What follows are excerpts from her Detroit entry:

I heard about Nora Coffey from my sister who knew a woman whom she had counseled. She believed ignoring Nora was the biggest mistake she ever made as she has had five more operations since.

During the two weeks prior to the protest I visited various facilities frequented by women (e.g. health clubs, hair salons, grocery stores, local libraries, churches, and Gilda's Club) and dropped off play announcements. I also distributed flyers by mail to numerous friends. Three times a week I would replenish the flyers and pamphlets in the women's locker room of the fitness center where I am a member. This really worked well as I was able to initiate conversations with other members.

One morning, in particular, a woman I approached with the HERS pamphlets refused to take them saying, "Hysterectomy - I know all about that. I already had mine and it was the best thing I ever did. I'm fine." Further questioning revealed her hysterectomy was due to fibroid tumors. Next I asked if she had been put on hormones. She answered, "Yes," so I asked if she developed breast cancer. She answered, "Yes, but it was caught early and I'm fine." She added that her husband was a doctor...

I made contact with media personnel in the Detroit area (newspapers and radio stations). I spoke to Mark Rosenthal, the producer of the Mitch Albom talk radio show on WJR760, and

was advised he could not publicize the protest
march at St. Joseph Mercy Hospital in Pontiac.
Station WWJ NewsRadio 95 and a few other stations agreed to announce it on their website.

I met with two female reporters at the Birmingham Eccentric Newspaper who were happy to
post a notice on their website and run a brief
article announcing the play, "Un Becoming,"
to take place at the Birmingham Community
House. Approximately 45 persons attended the
performance, and I was quite pleased. The post-
play discussion session with Nora Coffey and
Rick Schweikert, the playwright, was very lively.

As for the picketing at St. Joseph Mercy Oakland Hospital, the volunteers (including a few
husbands) handed out pamphlets, carried signs,
and spoke to passers by. One of the hospital employees entering the driveway told Alice (one
of the protestors) that she would have her removed from the sidewalk because she was picketing on private property. Alice responded that
the sidewalk is public property. No attempt was
made to remove her or the other protesters.

One morning when I was standing at the main
driveway entrance, a man in his forties pulled
up in a sports car. As I approached his vehicle
from the passenger's side with my sign and pamphlets he admonished me in an arrogant tone
saying, "What are you doing standing in front
of this hospital?" I must admit I was a bit taken
back. I replied that this was the perfect place to
stand because this hospital performed hysterectomies, some of which were likely unnecessary.
He yelled, "Who are you to decide that?" I said,
"I'm a patient and you don't give women the
full story." He said, "What do you mean? I'm an
OB-GYN and I run a pelvic pain clinic in Detroit
and women are begging for hysterectomies." I

stated, "You don't inform them of the adverse effects and alternatives to the procedure ahead of time." He said, "They sign a consent form." I said, "It's actually an *uninformed* consent form because women are not advised of the damage resulting from the surgery." Horns were blowing because he was blocking the driveway. As he pulled away, I placed the HERS brochure on the front passenger seat of his car, which he probably didn't appreciate.

The next day during the hospital lunch hour, I was approached by a doctor who said he was a general surgeon and very politely asked why we were picketing at this hospital. He stated that they don't perform unnecessary hysterectomies in St. Joseph's Hospital and he would report any unethical behavior. One of the other protesters was standing nearby and informed him of the unnecessary hysterectomy that his wife had been given at St. Joe's. He accepted our handouts and appeared interested in them. Most of the hospital personnel who spoke with us insisted that only necessary hysterectomies were performed, especially since this is a Catholic hospital.

Later in the week I was approached by a middle-aged woman who told me that her mother had a hysterectomy after 30 years of marriage and five children to prevent further pregnancies. Following it she was not the same person. After the surgery, her father divorced her mother. I gave her the HERS pamphlets. She looked them over and said, "Now I understand what happened to my mother." She asked for extra pamphlets to distribute to her co-workers.

During the week following the Michigan protest, I learned that a woman to whom I had given pamphlets had contacted the HERS Foundation to express her gratitude. The information she received from me was very timely in that one of her daughters was scheduled to have a hysterectomy. The daughter changed her mind. The woman also stated that her other two daughters had been considering hysterectomies and also changed their minds. This type of feedback really encouraged me to continue with the volunteer work in other cities.

We had a good turnout for the reading of *un becoming*. Rachael of DreamWeavers Theatre Troupe assembled a last-minute cast that did a fine job. In the talkback, someone said, "Is there anything we can do to actually stop unconsented hysterectomy once and for all?"

"We're working on a legislative solution," I said, "and soon we'll need everyone's help."

The conversation that Nora and I had almost two months earlier on the beach in Massachusetts continued off and on throughout the year. And in Detroit we began trying it out on the public. Politically, the country couldn't have been more divided, so we began asking protestors, "Would you change your vote from George Bush to John Kerry or from John Kerry to George Bush if the other guy vowed to work with HERS to end unconsented hysterectomy?"

One of them said, "If they worked with HERS, yes, I'd change my vote."

"Yes, I'd change my vote," another person said, "because millions of women can be saved with one simple law."

Later Sue and Brian would join our Full Disclosure Consent Campaign Committee to hold meetings with attorneys, scholars, civil rights experts, and other supporters to embark on a plan to end unconsented hysterectomy.

As with most readings of the play, there was one woman in the Detroit audience who said hysterectomy was the best thing she ever did, even after a roomful of women talked about how hysterectomy was the worst thing that was ever done to them. She and the others continued telling stories and asking questions long after we were supposed to leave the community center at the end of the night.

TWENTY-FIVE

The uterus and the cardiovascular advantage.

Burlington, Vermont—Nora W. Coffey

According to their website, "Approximately 2,200 deliveries are performed each year at Fletcher Allen and approximately 1,200 gynecologic surgical procedures are performed annually." Note how Fletcher Allen Health Care refers to deliveries as being "performed" by doctors, equating birth with other procedures doctors perform, rather than the natural function performed by the women who actually deliver babies. When you take away weekends and holidays, Fletcher Allen doctors perform about five gynecological surgeries each day and one gynecological surgery for every girl born there.

Mary Fletcher founded the hospital in 1876. In 1894, The Religious Hospitallers of St. Joseph founded the Fanny Allen Hospital, named after Frances Margaret Allen, daughter of Ethan Allen, the early American revolutionary who's sometimes called the "Father of Vermont." Both are now teaching hospitals "in alliance with the University of Vermont."[82]

Near the hospital, there wasn't a lot of foot traffic, so I went into town. I handed pamphlets out to disengaged passersby, most of whom took little interest in why I was there. At the end of the day, I headed to a restaurant I'd been to before on visits to Burlington, when my son lived there.

A man seated at the opposite end of the bar recommended the shrimp when he saw me scanning the menu. I asked if he'd

---

[82] http://www.fahc.org/gme/OBGYN/services.html.

eaten there before, and he said he had...every day for the last 20 years. It wasn't until then I noticed he was shelling a bowl of shrimp.

He asked about my t-shirt, with the *un becoming* logo and the Protest & Play schedule. When I told him why I was there his hands stopped and he stared down into the bowl of shrimp. "I own this place with my ex-wife," he said. "We're still good friends, but she had a hysterectomy four years after our son was born. After that, she said she couldn't be around people anymore. Now she's having some problems with her heart, but that's probably not related to the surgery," he said, like he knew I was about to tell him otherwise.

"If her uterus was removed but her ovaries weren't," I said, "she has a three times greater risk of heart disease. And if her ovaries were also removed, she has a seven times greater risk."

In his article "Prostacyclin From The Uterus And Woman's Cardiovascular Advantage," James D. Shelton says, "Prostacyclin emanating from the uterus is proposed as a major contributor to the reduced risk of coronary disease among women." He refers to the uterus as a "systemically active organ whose removal significantly increases subsequent risk of myocardial infarction."[83]

"And she's having trouble walking," he said. "Problems with her balance, I guess. You don't think that has anything to do with it, do you?"

"About 35% of hysterectomized women experience frequent dizziness after the surgery," I said. "And based on the women I've counseled who have nerve damage, it's likely she has femoral neuropathy. She may be having problems because the blood sup-

[83] Shelton, James D., "Prostacyclin From The Uterus And Woman's Cardiovascular Advantage," *Prostaglandins Leukotrienes and Medicine*, 1982.

ply to her uterus had to be severed to remove it, so the blood flow to her pelvis and legs is diminished."

An article titled "Nerve Injury At Abdominal Hysterectomy" by Kim Morgan and E. J. Thomas reports that "injury to the lateral femoral cutaneous nerve of the thigh following abdominal hysterectomy...appears to occur relatively frequently."[84] From my experience, "relatively frequently" is putting the problem quite mildly.

The owner of the restaurant continued running the business with his wife, he said, but she was rarely there. He often visited her, but their previous social life and sexual intimacy was gone. He never knew why, but now he realized it was the hysterectomy that had altered the course of their lives in so many ways. Neither had remarried. He said she did her best to be the mother her son needed her to be, but she was never the same.

It's unlikely there's anyone in this country whose life is untouched by hysterectomy. There's one degree of separation or less between each of us and someone who's been directly impacted by it.

Because I had the feeling it would be too overwhelming for him, I didn't offer him a HERS pamphlet. He didn't seem to need any further verification than his own experiences and our conversation. He softly said, "Thank you," and left.

In every election the public is reminded how we tend to vote with the issues that relate to basic survival and security. The newspaper looking up at me from the bar was dominated by stories related to the 2004 presidential race. I thought about how so many of the issues in this newspaper simply don't matter in the same way to the women and families whose lives have been shattered by hysterectomy.

[84] Morgan, Kim and Thomas, E. J., "Nerve Injury At Abdominal Hysterectomy," *British Journal of Obstetrics and Gynecology*, 1995.

TWENTY-SIX

Capitalizing on fear of "the C word."

Chicago, Illinois—Nora W. Coffey

Men are more likely to get cancer than women.[85] Men develop prostate cancer, testicular cancer, penile cancer, breast cancer, and male infertility is becoming extremely profitable for the medical industrial complex, but while most cities have women's hospitals, I'm not aware of one men's hospital. In spite of the billions of dollars pumped into cancer research, cancer rates have been fairly stable for both sexes for more than 30 years.[86] And yet the female organs are removed from more than $1/3^{rd}$ of all women in this country by the age of 60, while the rate of male organ removal is almost non-existent.

Many women who contact HERS for physician referrals prefer female gynecologists. They believe that a woman wouldn't recommend an unnecessary hysterectomy and will understand why they want to keep their uterus and ovaries. Others go so far as to attribute the overuse of hysterectomy to the fact that medicine is male-dominated. But several studies, such as "The impact of nonclinical factors on practice variations: the case of hysterectomies," indicate otherwise. "Female physicians," the study points out, "are more likely than their male counterparts to perform a hysterectomy."[87]

---

[85] Pal, Somnath Pal, "Men Lead Women In Cancer Incidence," *U.S. Pharmacist*, Volume 23:5.
[86] Ibid.
[87] Geller, S. E. et al, "The impact of nonclinical factors on practice variations: the case of hysterectomies," *Health Services Research*, February 1996.

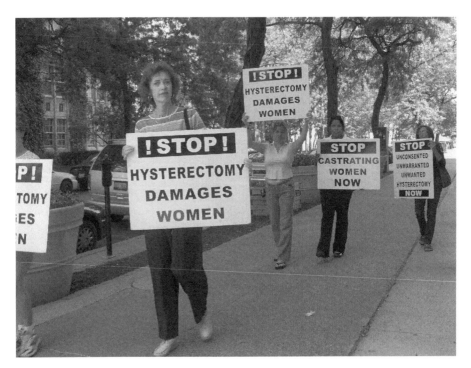

The Prentice Women's Hospital in Chicago (affiliated with Northwestern University's Feinberg School of Medicine) is, according to their website, "dedicated exclusively to women's health issues... here for you at all stages of your life."[88] I entered "hysterectomy" into the search box on Prentice's homepage. While Prentice may list the things they believe women should know about hysterectomy, their information is incomplete, and some of it is incorrect and potentially damaging. They fail to provide even the most basic information.

Under the heading "Patient Education," visitors are provided with "Total Vaginal Hysterectomy and Removal of the Ovaries (Laparoscopic): Patient Discharge Instructions," in which Prentice states, "if you feel good and are well-rested, sexual activity may

---

[88] http://prentice.nmh.org/nmh/prentice/main.htm.

be resumed."[89] By means of comparison, Louisiana Senate Bill 144, Act 441 allows for repeat male sex offenders to be castrated. If castration (the medical term for removal of either the testicles or ovaries) has the desired effect on male sex offenders, how is it that Prentice and Northwestern Memorial Hospital fail to mention that removal of the gonads also destroys female sexuality? Are women expected to resume sexual activity in Illinois after castration, whereas male sex offenders are castrated in Louisiana to prevent that very thing from ever happening again?

This would be the second protest for Joan, who organized the Detroit protest. Here's her account of her experiences at the Prentice Women's Hospital:

> Many of the medical people completely ignored us when they saw our signs and were, in fact, rude and refused to accept the brochures. The few that did engage in conversation were very argumentative, including a pre-med student who was very stubborn and would not recognize the possibility that hysterectomies had adverse effects. Surprisingly, one young student approached Nora and actually asked her for a pamphlet saying his mother had recently had the surgery and was having problems. I asked another young man who refused my handout if he was a student at Northwestern and he said Yes. Next I asked what school he attended and he replied the law school. After I told him my husband was a lawyer he accepted my handout. Apparently that gave me credibility in his mind.

Some of the protestors were surprised by the response from the medical students, but I expected it. We met only a few

---

[89] http://www.nmh.org/nmh/pdf/pated/totalhyst-abdischarge07.pdf.

who weren't rude. Here's a quote from Robert Mendelsohn's *MALePRACTICE*:

> ... Medical schools teach a great deal of pro-
> fessional misconduct, neatly cloaked in pious
> rhetoric. The character and behavior of the stu-
> dents are altered by it. You—the patient—pay
> the always costly and sometimes mortal price.
> That's why I am unwilling to let anyone in the
> medical profession, including myself, off the
> hook.

Mendelson also urges us to avoid teaching hospitals for surgery:

> Enter one, and they'll get their on-the-job train-
> ing practicing on you... Obviously, there is a
> point at which every surgical resident must take
> his first slice at a nice, warm belly, but do you re-
> ally want it to be the one that belongs to you?[90]

A security guard came out to speak with us because we set our boxes of materials on hospital property. I expected the worst, but then he said rather meekly, "Why are you protesting?" I gave him a pamphlet, which he read as he walked away. He didn't bothered us again.

A FedEx driver screeched to a stop, got out of the truck, grabbed a pamphlet, then got back in and raced away. Many women took a pamphlet from us, read it cover-to-cover, and then walked beside us throughout the protest talking about the issues.

One medical student sheepishly took a pamphlet from me as the other students he was with laughed and made snide remarks. I said, "I hope you're not the only student here who's brave enough to become educated." When the others moved on, he told

---

[90] Mendelsohn, Robert S., *MALePRACTICE: How Doctors Manipulate Women*, Contemporary Books, 1981.

me his mother was hysterectomized and was never the same again. He was aware of how the surgery changed her and was grateful to finally know why.

I met with my aunt in Chicago. She'd had a hysterectomy a few years earlier. She's an excellent writer, documentary filmmaker, astute observer, crossword puzzle master, and one of my best critics. I count on her truthful opinions, always accompanied by a large dose of unerring encouragement and support. I wasn't prepared for how much she had changed in the few years since I saw her last. All her life she was slim, but now, although she was still small on top, her hips were a bit wide. At dinner she said it wasn't until we spoke that she associated her second heart attack and broken hip with having undergone a hysterectomy. After that visit, she had another heart attack and another surgery that she barely survived.

TWENTY-SEVEN

Sex improved by removing sex organs?

Bismarck, North Dakota—Nora W. Coffey

Requiring citizens to obtain a permit to protest flies in the face of the First Amendment rights guaranteed by the U.S. Constitution. In Bismarck, not only did we need a permit, they also required a notarized signature on the permit application to "indemnify and hold harmless the city of Bismarck."

The notion of a hold-harmless agreement for a peaceful protest was ludicrous. When the permit application arrived in the mail, it reminded me of the hospital consent forms, which also asked me to sign away my most basic rights.

Before I signed this waiver, I requested and received a copy of the pertinent city ordinance. I didn't like it, but I was now in a position to make an informed decision whether or not to sign Bismarck's hold harmless agreement.

Initially I refused, but it became clear that our protest at Medcenter One Health Systems would be considered illegal without it. So in front of the required notary, I wrote my objection directly onto the protest application: "Signed against my better judgment. The city holds the permit hostage. It is tantamount to blackmail."

After we received the permit, Medcenter One Health Systems sent a letter to Deborah Ness, Chief of Police, requesting that we "choose a less congested area" for our protest. James Cooper, President/CBO of the medical center, said he was "concerned with this protest in terms of safety."[91] We were also concerned about safety—not so much for the minor traffic congestion our protest would cause outside Medcenter One, but for the women who might find themselves *inside* the hospital, in need of our help.

The unreasonable permit process and attempted intervention by the hospital administrator left me with low expectations, but I was pleasantly surprised with Bismarck, where the North Dakota license plates beckon visitors to "discover the spirit" in The Peace Garden State.

I was interviewed by the local Fox and ABC affiliates. The interviewer from ABC was very good. A graduate of Columbia, she didn't seem out of her element covering a protest about a serious topic. It was clearly odd for her and her crew to interview a woman in Bismarck, protesting alone on the side of an 8-lane road. They were impressed and moved by the number of people who came to show their support for HERS. Both interviews aired more than once, which probably accounted for the increase in visitors to the protest site over the next few days. A lot of older people honked and waved as they drove by, some stopping to tell me to "be careful."

Like Rapid City, Bismarck was dusty, and I felt like the walls of my hotel room were closing in on me. I drove out into the country until I was too tired to stay awake and pulled over to sleep. It was beautiful country, and I felt at ease with the wide-open sky above me.

The next day I found a good restaurant. I sat in the middle of the patio. A man and a woman sat together at a table at one

---

[91] Cooper, James, Medcenter One Health Systems, a letter to Deborah Ness, Bismarck Chief of Police, faxed from the City of Bismarck to the HERS Foundation, September 10, 2004.

end of the patio, two men sat at the other end. I tried to tune out what the two men were saying, but one of them was very loud, their conversation having something to do with corporate medicine. Finally, when I realized I wouldn't be able to drown them out with my own thoughts, I asked them what they did there in Bismarck.

The louder one was morbidly obese and had a thick accent. He chewed on a cigar, the living picture of poor health. He said he was from the Dominican Republic and was there "to fill in at the hospital." The other one looked like a military man—very rigid in conversation and body language. He elaborated a bit, saying, "We're part of a business that hires retired military doctors to fill in around the country…to plug holes when a doctor's on vacation or the hospital's between doctors."

"So you fill-in in your area of specialty anywhere you're called?"

"No," he said dismissively, "we do whatever's needed. In any department."

"If a pulmonary surgeon's on vacation you fill in, even if that's not your specialty?" I asked.

"Sure. Whatever's needed." Then he asked, "And now, what're *you* doing here?"

I told them, and they seemed unopposed to the need for a protest against unconsented hysterectomy. The one with the stiff mannerisms gave me his card—"Frank L. Johnson, M.D., Colonel, USAF, MC (Retired)."

The doctor from the Dominican Republic sat down at my table uninvited. He said he wanted to talk about "this issue of unnecessary hysterectomy. I think all the women who have it need it," he said, "and it improves the lives of the women who have it."

"So tell me exactly how you think women are improved by having their sex organs removed," I said.

"Well," he exclaimed, "they still have sex organs!"

"And if a surgeon removed your penis and testicles, you'd still have sex organs."

The discussion went back and forth that way. I pointed out to them that the military provides 100% disability for removal of the uterus and ovaries for 6 months after the surgery, and 50% disability for life.[92] Bit by bit, I laid out the problem of hysterectomy, until eventually he agreed hysterectomy is a damaging surgery. In spite of his acknowledgement, he attempted to turn the conversation back to talking about ways that hysterectomy might improve a woman's life, or as he put it, "the problems it solves."

"Except in about 2% of hysterectomies," I said, "there are more conservative treatment options. Would you take the same approach with male sex organs or with any other part of the body? No, of course not. So why are female organs any different?"

The conversation seemed to end there. As a closing comment, I said no matter how badly a hysterectomy consent law is needed, nothing would be done to change the laws in the current political climate. Suddenly, the colonel became irritated. He said he was a fervent supporter of the Bush administration. They were Republicans who had served in the military and their company was owned by retired military doctors. "And this war in Iraq is necessary!" he said.

I was inclined to remind him that I had said nothing about Bush or the war. I merely said that the problem of a lack of

---

[92] Social Security Disability Benefits Reform Act of 1984, Public Law 98-460, Section 4.116, Diagnostic Code 7617.

informed consent relative to hysterectomy isn't likely to go away in the current political climate, which includes Independents and Democrats, as well as Republicans. But before I could do so, the man sitting with the woman at the other table spoke for the first time, saying he agreed with the retired military doctors, because he too supported the Bush administration.

I was dumbfounded. They knew nothing about my political affiliation or how I felt about anything going on in the Middle East. So I returned to my own thoughts, which is what I sought by sitting at a table set off from the others.

The wind picked up again, and our plates were covered with another fine layer of dust. The obese doctor went on talking loudly, and the couple sat there eating without a word between them.

TWENTY-EIGHT

Twice as healthy with half as much medicine.

Omaha, Nebraska—Rick Schweikert

The University of Nebraska Medical Center, the site of our Nebraska protest, is located just a half mile's drive south down 41st Street from where I grew up. And the Shelterbelt Theatre, where *un becoming* would be performed, is located on California Street, about a mile east of my childhood home.

The *Omaha World Herald* and *The Reader* both published articles about the Protest & Play. Because of those articles and the familiar faces of family and friends, we had a full house. The reading, directed by Daena Schweiger was well received and was followed by a lively talkback.

Probably because I knew some of the people in the audience, they were more interested in talking about the play and HERS than their own experiences with hysterectomy. Mr. Watson, who was active in our neighborhood when I was a kid, said he was impressed that Nora recognized the potential of theater to educate the public. We also talked a lot about the need to put information back into informed consent. I quoted Ivan Illich's book *Limits to Medicine*, where he says, "The medical establishment has become a major threat to health."[93] Someone else in the audience said, "We'd all probably be twice as healthy with half as much medicine." But then my niece Ashley spoke up.

Ashley had been fighting some potentially fatal health problems all her life. She wanted to let everyone know that without

---

[93] Illich, Ivan, *Limits to Medicine*, Marion Boyars, 1976.

specialists at the Mayo Clinic, she might've died. I was proud of her for being bold enough to speak out about her own experiences when it ran contrary to the discussion. Nora said, "The bad doesn't make the good worse, and the good doesn't make the bad better."

In 2005, "operations on the female genital organs" (1,967,000) and "obstetrical procedures" (6,858,000, almost all of which were the result of the medicalization of pregnancy and birthing, such as doctor-induced and doctor-accelerated delivery) represented about 20% of all procedures performed on both women and men in "non-federal" U.S. hospitals.[94] Some doctors do good work, I told Ashley, but there are enough gynecologists performing unwarranted, damaging procedures on women to warrant immediate action.

The nearest hospital to my childhood home was the Bishop Clarkson Memorial Hospital, which later became the University of Nebraska Medical Center. I could never have guessed that one day I'd be protesting against unconsented hysterectomy on these familiar streets. Anna from Denver was also born in Omaha, and we knew from the sign-up list we'd have a good turnout. Anna's husband came too. He sat across the street at a bus stop taking pictures of the protest.

Early on a security guard came out to speak with us. His uniform hung from him like a cheap costume, and he couldn't have been less intimidating. "They heard you'd be here," he said, "so they sent me out to tell you it's okay for you to use the facilities."

"Thanks," I said.

"Sure. Just don't bring any of your stuff inside."

Just then a young man who didn't look old enough to be driving pulled over to the curb and waved for me to come to him.

[94] "Advance Data No. 385, United States 2005," *CDC*, July 12, 2007.

Speaking through his car window, I told him about HERS and the protest.

"They do that at this hospital too?" he asked, as he threw the car into park.

"At every hospital where hysterectomies are performed," I said.

"Well, that's what killed my mom."

"How long ago?"

"About a year ago. She went in, but she didn't come out."

"I'm sorry to hear that."

"Well, except when they took her to the funeral home." He took a few pamphlets, saying, "I can give these to the girls at work." He shook my hand, but he didn't drive away. He just sat there, staring out his windshield. Finally, he put his foot on the brake and threw his car back into gear, saying, "They killed my mom," and he slowly drove off down 42nd Street.

Later, Nora and I went downtown to M's Pub for lunch with Brenda, Patti, and Anna. Nora asked them if they'd change their vote for President if the other candidate supported hysterectomy informed consent legislation. We were then just over a month away from the big election. Brenda said she'd change her vote from Bush to Kerry, but only if they worked with HERS to do it. Then Patti said she'd also change her vote, but her switch would be from Kerry to Bush. Anna said she wouldn't change her vote from Bush to Kerry based on this single issue, but it would make her "think more highly of Kerry if he did."

The next morning, the young man who stopped to talk with me the day before drove by the protest at the same time in the same direction, probably heading to work again. He waved and gave us the thumbs-up.

TWENTY-NINE

Dr. Bully, Dr. Friend, Dr. Slick

New York, New York—Nora W. Coffey

A large group of protestors met at the NYU Medical Center in midtown Manhattan, including Joan from Detroit and my fearless friend Sybil Shainwald, a longtime activist and dynamic attorney who's respected and admired the world over for her advocacy in women's health law.[95]

In most cities we did our best to stay off private property. But after Sybil greeted each protester, without missing a beat she took up a sign and strode across the driveway right up to the front door. I called after her, "Sybil, you can't go onto hospital property." She yelled back, "Watch me!" She handed out a lot of information before security convinced her to rejoin us on the sidewalk.

Joan pointed out that the morgue and coroner's office were located beside the hospital. "Ghoulishly appropriately next door," she said. "How convenient."

A lot of the hospital personnel took literature from us. Many of the nurses and staff were grateful for the information, and some took the time to tell us they supported our mission. Most of the doctors, though, were angry and abusive. One female gynecologist in particular argued angrily in defense of hysterectomy as she stormed by, unaccustomed to listening to anyone. She personified the arrogant attitude of doctors who think they know everything, and we laypeople should do as we're told.

---

[95] "Sybil Shainwald is the first woman ever to receive the [New York Law School] President's Medal of Honor." *Alumni Connections*, New York Law School, May 2007.

Counseling women all day and hearing about their experiences with doctors, I divide hysterectomizing gynecologists into three basic personality types. First are the Bully gynecologists—the type that trivializes your questions and laughs at your concerns, making you feel stupid and insignificant. Next are the Good Friend gynecologists—the sensitive type that says, "Trust me, I have your best interests at heart. This is what I'd do if you were my own wife or daughter." The Good Friend gynecologists lull you into a false sense of security over a period of years, bonding with you through your pregnancy and birthing experience, pretending to be a friend of the family until they get you into the operating room…and then the friendship's over. Finally, there are the Slick gynecologists—tall, dark, and good looking, their attraction to you is so palpable you believe they're taking special care of you because they'd never hurt someone they're attracted to.

Women who are hysterectomized by Bully are generally angry when they call HERS. But they're often more angry at themselves for not standing up to the bully than they are at the doctor. Women who are hysterectomized by the other two types usually go back to the gynecologist to tell them that something must've gone wrong, because they have all these problems. When women tell Good Friend or Slick they have a loss of sexual feeling and don't feel like themselves anymore, that their vitality and interest in life is gone, Friend and Slick say, "I've never heard any of that before." Because women believe and trust doctors, they sometimes feel betrayed. Others are less comfortable with the idea that the deception was deliberate. They characterize it as "a mistake," as if it was something the doctor wouldn't have done if they realized it was going to cause problems.

Most women who are hysterectomized by a female doctor have a difficult time believing that a woman doctor would do this to another woman. Nor can they believe that a friend would do this to a friend or that an attractive doctor would do this to a sexy, sensual woman. But now Friend no longer treats her like a friend. And Slick doesn't flirt with her anymore.

We didn't meet Slick or Friend at our protests, we only met Bully. They might seem slick and friendly inside the hospital or while examining you, but on the sidewalk, confronted by protestors, almost every gynecologist we met was an arrogant and angry bully.

One of the protestors was a registered nurse with nerve damage and chronic pain. After she was hysterectomized she underwent four additional surgeries and was treated for numerous infections. "Take it from a nurse who's worked in many different hospitals for a whole lot of years," she said, "they're all dangerous places."

Each time a protestor returned to get more pamphlets, there was another story to tell from the field, like the protestor who met a woman who was a senior auditor of a pharmaceutical company before she was, as she put it, "fired for finding too much fault with some of their products."

Across the street I noticed a woman with a cane leaning against a signpost. After a while she motioned for me to cross the street. "You should stand over here with all of these doctors and medical students," she said. I took her advice, and she silently watched me work. Finally she said, "Can I have one of those?" I handed her a pamphlet, and she read it cover to cover. A few minutes later I looked over and she had tears streaming down her face. When she noticed I was looking at her, she held out her arm for a taxi. One immediately pulled over and she was gone.

The wake-up call for hysterectomy was no different here than it was anywhere else. We got the same looks from people in New York as we did in Anchorage. A taxi driver stopped at the light on 31st Street. I handed a pamphlet to his passenger, and like a shot they were off, the passenger riding down 3rd Avenue reading our pamphlet. There was a long line of taxis waiting near the hospital entrance. As I walked past them with my sign, about half of them leaned over the passenger side with an outstretched hand to take a pamphlet.

Most of the people we came in contact with in New York were receptive to our message. It wasn't at all the cold-hearted city of its reputation. Almost to a fault, everyone we met was warm, welcoming, and eager for information.

THIRTY

"For mom and apple pie."

Minneapolis, Minnesota—Rick Schweikert

When I was in Omaha with the protest, I asked my dad why he thought U.S. soldiers were still in Iraq two years after capturing Saddam Hussein and establishing regime change. He was a World War II vet, so he answered me with the slogan of soldiers in his generation—"For mom and apple pie." Later, when I was quoted in the Omaha press about the HERS protest, he asked me why I was "wasting my time protesting with a bunch of leftwing radicals." My answer was, "Only half of them are leftwing radicals. The other half are rightwing radicals. But I guess we're doing it for mom and apple pie."

Dad felt the need to label himself a conservative and me a liberal. I don't like either, but if a radical is someone who speaks out for women like my mother, my wife, my sisters, and my daughter, then maybe we need more radicals.

We picked up Joan from her Minneapolis hotel to join us at the Hennepin County Medical Center protest. In spite of debilitating physical limitations and great personal expense, she'd be out there once again educating women far from home. When Nora saw her she said, "There's a woman with true grit."

Although Nora downplays the praise she gets from women, countless women approached the protest asking, "Are you Nora Coffey? You saved my life." One of them was an attorney specializing in engineering and environmental law. She told Joan she consulted 20 doctors before finding one who'd perform a myomectomy. The previous 19 either lacked the skill or the incentive to do anything other than a hysterectomy, but in her case persistence paid off.

Four of the other protesters were needlessly hysterectomized. One of them knew right away that she didn't need the surgery because the same symptoms before the surgery got worse afterwards. It was her gallbladder that should've been removed, not her uterus. Now she couldn't work, and she was worried about her future.

In Minneapolis, we had one family with three generations of protesters. Bonnie brought her daughter and granddaughter to the protest. She said she'd change her vote from Bush to Kerry, if Kerry supported the HERS mandate.

Bonnie said she was hysterectomized for minor pains in her side. The doctor bullied her into the surgery because, he said, her ovaries were a potential breeding ground for cancer. She searched for an attorney to file a hysterectomy lawsuit, but none of them would take it because they couldn't find an expert willing to testify as a witness. She then wrote to the Medical Board, but they refused to take action, she said.

Bonnie's daughter said her mother had always been the life of the party, but after the surgery she was distant and depressed. "Now I live to keep my daughter and granddaughter out of the operating room," Bonnie told me.

After the protests were underway, Nora usually wandered off. Sometimes she papered the hospital parking garage or the gynecology department. Today Nora had her sights set on papering the cars in the church parking lot across the street.

Before long, a woman flew out of the rear door of the church. She took a pamphlet out from under the windshield wiper of the first car and crossed the street, yelling, "Who put these here?!"

"I did," Nora said.

The woman's entire body trembled when she said, "You can't do that! You have no right." When we didn't respond, she said with tears in her eyes, "You'll have to remove them all. Now!"

But Nora calmly said, "No. We're not going to remove them."

"If you won't remove them, I will, and they're all going into the garbage."

"I hope you won't do that," Nora said quietly, "but you should do whatever you have to."

The woman returned across the street and began ripping pamphlets from under windshield wipers. After a few cars she slowed down and looked over at us. She yelled something we couldn't make out, and then she went back inside, snatching the pamphlets from a few more cars as she went.

Soon church began letting out. One by one they took the pamphlets from their windshields and got into their cars. Many of them sat there reading them before they started their engines. Once they did, some of them pulled over to talk with us. Others waved or gave us the usual thumbs-up. One couple sat reading the pamphlet a long time before driving off. They were so engrossed in the information they ran a red light and almost caused an accident.

On another one of Nora's excursions, she met a woman sitting on a concrete bench between the hospital and a clinic. "She looked disheveled and sad," Nora said, "and she sat there motionless, nothing moving but her eyes as she watched me walk by with a

'Hysterectomy Damages Women' sign." Nora gave her a pamphlet, and the woman said, "So, that's what happened to me, huh?" She went on to say that she was in constant pain and had to wear adult diapers because of urinary incontinence. She was on Medicaid, and no one told her that her problems were related to the surgery. "I got hooked on drugs and alcohol to kill the pain," she said.

The Minneapolis reading of *un becoming* was held at The Playwright's Center after the first day of the protest, under the direction of my friend Bob Marion, who also joined us at the Milwaukee protest. In the play the character Megan Ridge, the doctor's daughter, makes an origami fortune-teller for Emma Douglas, the main protagonist. Later Emma teaches her friend John Tracey how to use it. In Minneapolis, Megan was played by 11-year-old Sarah Beaumont. When I asked Sarah to make a fortune-teller for the reading, these are the answers she wrote on the inside flaps of the fortune-teller:

1. something bad is going to happen to you
2. you like to do the foodley, foodley shoo with your toodley, toodley coo today
3. don't look back because I'm behind you
4. today you will be a happy, dappy yapper? Eat me!

During the performance Todd (playing the role of John) lifted the flap to get the answer for Carole (Sarah's mom, playing Emma), and showed it to her. Carole was so surprised by answer #2 her face flushed, which was perfect for her role. She was then supposed to crumple up the fortune-teller and toss it. Instead, she opened another answer, as if to get a second opinion, which no one had done before, but she was even more surprised by what

Sarah had written there for answer #4. She finally sat down and read the other two answers.

After the play Sarah marched over with a scowl and punched me on the arm, saying, "He made me do it!" Carole was close behind, and she punched me too.

"What was that for?" I asked. "It was one of the best Scene Thirteens of the year!"

THIRTY-ONE

Female Anatomy 101.

Billings, Montana—Nora W. Coffey

My first night in Billings I heard gunshots. I went to the window of my hotel room and saw the police converge. Detectives gathered evidence and took photos of the crime scene, while a crowd gathered to watch the painstaking effort to extract the victim from the car. After a while others rushed in to identify the body. A woman sobbed.

With that introduction to the city, our Montana protest began the next day. The Deaconess Billings Clinic was isolated with little pedestrian activity. It was a cold day, so we had to keep moving. Because of the limited foot traffic, we focused on distributing materials to people driving by in cars, but the drivers were less than receptive.

After a while a hospital representative came out to speak with us, asking quite formally if we'd please stop protesting in front of their hospital. Because of the cold weather I knew we wouldn't be out there much longer, but I didn't want to give him any indication that we might be persuaded to go away, so I said, "I understand how you feel, but we have no intention of leaving." Suddenly the formalities and courtesies vanished. He turned on his heel, yelling, "The authorities will soon be paying you a visit!"

That evening I had dinner at the restaurant where the shooting victim from the night before had worked in the kitchen. I didn't expect the restaurant to be open, but it was just like any other day.

Bernadette (name changed for confidentiality), the Billings protest coordinator, took me to her favorite rodeo. Children broncobusters were the opening bill. Watching children get strapped to beasts only to be violently bucked off was one of the more unusual experiences of the Protest & Play year. Their mothers ran out into the corral, scooped up their battered children, and then tended to their wounds as the next child was strapped on.

Bernadette attended the Billings protest hoping she'd be able to confront the doctor who hysterectomized her and learn about a cure for her post-operative problems. She thought maybe there was something I hadn't told her about during counseling that I could share with her at the protest.

It's always disheartening for women to discover there's no "cure" for the damage caused by hysterectomy. Although the damage is irreversible, many women do get some degree of relief by taking a hormone called dehydroepiandrosterone (DHEA). DHEA is produced by the ovaries in a very small quantity, but it's extremely important because it's a precursor to the production of androgens, such as testosterone. Androgens help maintain energy, weight, muscle tissue, collagen (a major fibrous protein in bones, skin, cartilage, and connective tissue), and they play a part in the firing of synapses in the brain, which in turn influence memory and cognition. These powerful hormones also have a positive effect on sleep and dreaming.

Women who take DHEA consistently report getting some degree of relief from joint pain, severe dry eyes, hair loss, insomnia, loss of memory, and impaired cognition. It's not a magic bullet cure, but with DHEA many hysterectomized women say they have less trouble getting out of bed in the morning, their legs don't feel like lead, they have memory and cognition improvement, and a better quality of sleep. It's most effective when taken in the morning, but when taken at night it can have the opposite effect and interfere with sleep. The most common side effects they report are oily skin and facial hair.

One woman who received counseling from HERS retired early from her job as a professor because of short-term memory loss after the surgery. But with DHEA she had such significant improvement she said she may not have retired if she had found it earlier. Another woman stopped driving because of severe dry eyes, but with DHEA the condition improved enough for her to be able to drive again.

DHEA is packaged in 5mg to 200mg dosages—over 200mg requires a prescription. Individual tolerance to it varies enormously and may change over time. Some women need only 5mg, while others take 600mg or more a day. A cautious approach would be to take 15mg/day for two weeks. If there's no improvement in symptoms, it can be increased until some relief is experienced. Often women know they have found the optimal amount when their skin becomes somewhat oily and they develop pimples, but these reactions usually disappear in a few weeks.

Many women report that over-the-counter androgens are not as effective as those that are produced by a reputable compounding pharmacy. Because of the way DHEA is processed, variations in potency may occur. If it's over-processed, for example, it can result in decreased potency. Also, capsules seem to be more effective than tablets. Less than 200mg of DHEA is considered over-the-counter so pharmacies are permitted to sell it without a prescription. Two pharmacies that women report they've received consistently good DHEA capsules from are Apothécure in Dallas, Texas and the Women's International Pharmacy in Madison, Wisconsin.

The doctor who hysterectomized Bernadette in Billings never mentioned DHEA to her. She found it through her own research. Although she experienced some relief from some of her symptoms, she realized it wasn't a cure. Nor did the doctor come out of the hospital during the protest. As both realizations washed over her, she became very sad. "Why do people do this to each other?" she asked. None of my answers was satisfactory. "So what, this just doesn't ever end and doctors go on doing this to women forever and nobody cares?"

After the protest we drove outside the city. Bernadette was my tour guide to some breathtaking Rocky Mountain vistas. We drove up the long entrance of a ski resort until we came to a locked gate, but instead of turning around and heading back she pulled on the emergency brake, got out, and started rummaging around in a compartment behind the seat. When she returned she was holding a rifle.

"I carry this around just in case," she said.

I understood her meaning immediately, but it took a while to find the words. "If you kill the doctor," I said, "you'll make a martyr out of him."

"I know. I don't want that, that's for sure."

Then we talked about not leaving suicide as a legacy for her children. "No one could ever mother your children the same way you do," I said.

We drove to a tiny town with five bars in two blocks and bantered with the bartender as Bernadette drank herself numb.

She said, "I signed the consent form, but I didn't know what I was agreeing to. Nobody knows what this is, right, until it's too late?"

Hysterectomy is unconsented unless women are provided with:

- a female anatomy lesson
- information about the functions of the female organs
- information about the alternatives in treatment—including no treatment—and the risks of those alternatives
- information about the well-documented adverse effects of hysterectomy and female castration
- a simple description of what is cut, sutured, and repositioned during the surgery, and the consequences of severing the nerves, ligaments, and blood supply that attach to the uterus

It's grossly negligent that hospitals and doctors fail to provide this information to women. I have yet to find one hospital that does. What we found on the Protest & Play tour was doctors, hospital administrators, and websites repeating the same misleading and false information.

To Err Is Human, a report by the Institute of Medicine on the quality of healthcare in the U.S., was shocking to some but not a surprise to others. Among the findings is the following:

> At least 44,000 Americans die each year as a result of medical errors. The results of the New York Study suggest the number may be as high as 98,000. Even when using the lower estimate, deaths due to medical errors exceed the number attributable to the 8th-leading cause of death. More people die in a given year as a result of medical errors than from motor vehicle

accidents (43,458), breast cancer (42,297), or AIDS (16,516).[96]

Research by Gary Null, PhD and others paints an even gloomier picture:

> ...American medicine frequently causes more harm than good. The number of people having in-hospital, adverse drug reactions (ADR) to prescribed medicine is 2.2 million. Dr. Richard Besser, of the CDC, in 1995, said the number of unnecessary antibiotics prescribed annually for viral infections was 20 million... The number of unnecessary medical and surgical procedures performed annually is 7.5 million. The number of people exposed to unnecessary hospitalization annually is 8.9 million. The total number of iatrogenic deaths shown in the following table is 783,936. It is evident that the American medical system is the leading cause of death and injury in the United States.[97]

Other sources put the number of iatrogenic deaths in the U.S. somewhere between 120,000 to 180,000 each year.

Referring to an article he read on naturalnews.com,[98] a protestor in Detroit who was an avid hunter put it this way:

> There are more than 80 million gun owners in America and 1,500 accidental gun-related deaths each year, which comes out to .0000188 accidental deaths per gun owner. There are over 700,000 doctors in America and more than 120,000 reported deaths due to doctor error or

---

[96] Kohn, Linda T., Corrigan, Janet M., and Donaldson, Molla S., Editors, *To Err is Human: Building a Safer Health System*, Institute of Medicine Committee on Quality of Health Care in America, National Academy Press, 2000.

[97] Null, Gary et al, *Death by Medicine*, Nutrition Institute of America, 2003.

[98] "Doctors kill more people than guns: urban legend or fact?" Ben Kage, *Natural News Network*, November 30, 2006.

negligence, which comes out to .171 accidental deaths per doctor. Therefore, doctors are 9,000 times more likely to kill you than a gun owner.

In 1911, Reverend F. W. Herzberger made a case for forming an organization of nurses to become trained "in the great fields of missions and charities." Some time later the Lutheran Deaconess Association was founded because, as Herzberger said, "We need visiting nurses who can go into the hovels of the poor in our large cities or into the isolated homes in the countryside, especially when epidemics are abroad, and there nurse and comfort the sick and dying."[99] The Deaconess Billings Clinic has come a long way since those days of caring for the sick in the "hovels of the poor."

Information about hysterectomy on the Deaconness website is incomplete and contains potentially dangerous, erroneous information. Regarding the effects of hysterectomy on sexual experience, in a section titled "Sexual concerns following a hysterectomy," it says:

> Women who report decreased sexual enjoyment following a hysterectomy often do not have support from their sex partner. Before your surgery, talk with your partner about your concerns about sex following your hysterectomy. Find out about your partner's feelings…[100]

But no matter how supportive a woman's sex partner might be, she can't experience uterine orgasm without a uterus. Talking with her partner about her feelings won't make uterine orgasm possible anymore than talking with a man with no penis will help him get an erection.

---

[99] http://www.lifeoftheworld.com/lotw/article.php?a_num=6&m_num=2&m_vol=8.
[100] http://www.billingsclinic.com/body.cfm?xyzpdqabc=0&id=416&action=detail&AE ProductID=HW_Knowledgebase&AEArticleID=tv1991.

238 The H Word

Although they reference two studies, they fail to mention others that contradict the statements made on their website, such as the groundbreaking research by Alfred Kinsey known as *The Kinsey Report,* and the widely-respected book *Human Sexual Response* by William Masters and Virginia Johnson, which has been in continuous publication since 1966 and has been translated into more than 30 languages. Nor could we find a Deaconness reference to "Effect of Hysterectomy, Oophorectomy and Estrogen Therapy on Libido," which says, "The significant finding of the present study is the high incidence of decreased or absent libido in all groups of patients having undergone the operation of hysterectomy, irrespective of whether the ovaries had been conserved or not."[101] Or "Sexual Response After Hysterectomy-Oophorectomy: Recent Studies and Reconsideration of Psychogenesis," which demonstrates that dismissing the loss of sexual pleasure is "no longer tenable in the light of current physiologic knowledge of female anatomy."[102]

It's convenient for doctors and hospitals to dismiss sexual pleasure in women and say there's "no loss" or only the "possibility of sexual loss." Some women tell HERS they never enjoyed sex prior to surgery. A woman in Billings asked me, "I never had an orgasm before my hysterectomy, does this mean I never will?"

The discomfort and embarrassment that many people feel when talking about sex make it nearly impossible for some women to speak about the loss of sexual feeling, except in euphemisms.

---

[101] Utian, Wulf H., "Effect of Hysterectomy, Oophorectomy and Estrogen Therapy on Libido," *International Journal of Gynecology and Obstetrics*, 1975.
[102] Zussman, L. et al, "Sexual Response After Hysterectomy-Oophorectomy: Recent Studies and Reconsideration of Psychogenesis," *American Journal of Obstetrics and Gynecology*, 1981.

Many women have told us, "I don't feel anything down there anymore." Others say they feel "numb between the legs." Although many women do talk openly about the loss of sexual feeling, many who can talk about it choose not to because no one wants to be known as asexual. Many women have never told anyone except a HERS counselor that they have a loss of sexual feeling and fake orgasms. They live in fear that their partners will find out and won't enjoy sex with them and will look outside of their relationship to fill their sexual needs.

It's not surprising that women are unaware of any of this prior to surgery. The anatomical drawing that Deaconess offers on their website is labeled the "reproductive system." The implication is that they're only reproductive organs, so women who aren't planning to have a baby don't need them. Many doctors commonly refer to the uterus as a "baby bag," which is a dangerous characterization.

What's needed is a female anatomy lesson. Rick agreed, and he asked me where we could get one.

"I don't think one exists," I said. "Not one that's specific to women who're told they need a hysterectomy. But I give anatomy lessons to women every day."

"You give women an anatomy lesson every day? So, what do you tell them?" he asked.

He of course had overheard my anatomy lesson before in bits and pieces, and he knew most of what I told him, but it was the first time that I laid it all out for him:

> The uterus is a powerful muscle located in the lower pelvis. Our first awareness of the uterus is when we are taught that it is where a baby develops during pregnancy. Later we are taught

about menstruation, conception, and contraception. But that is generally where the education about the functions of the uterus ends. In fact, pregnancy is just one of the many functions of the uterus.

The uterus is a hormone-responsive reproductive sex organ that supports the bladder and the bowel. The bladder sits in front of the uterus, and the bowel sits behind it. The uterus separates them and helps keep the bladder in its natural position above the pubic bone and the bowel in its natural configuration behind the uterus.

The uterus is continuous with the cervix, which is continuous with the vagina, much in the way that your head is continuous with your neck, which is continuous with your shoulders. When the uterus is removed, the cervix is usually removed as well.

The uterus is attached to broad bands of ligaments, bundles of nerves, and networks of arteries and veins. Regardless of whether the hysterectomy is "total" or "partial," all of the ligaments, nerves, and blood supply attached to the uterus must be severed to remove it.

The round ligaments, cardinal ligaments, broad ligaments, and uterosacral ligaments that attach to the uterus provide structural integrity and support to the pelvic bones and the pelvic organs. When those ligaments are severed, women experience an unnatural shifting of the bones and organs inside the pelvis.

The severing of the ligaments permits the pelvic bones to move and widen, affecting the hips, lower back, and skeletal structure. The displacement of the pelvic bones results in compression of the spine. Women report that as the spine compresses, the rib cage gradually drifts down until it sits directly on the hip bones. This compression is the reason why hysterectomized women have protruding bellies and little or no waist.

Weakening of the pelvic floor and a loss of feeling from the severing of pelvic nerves may result in urinary incontinence (an inability to control urination), chronic constipation, or fecal incontinence (leakage and inability to control stool).

Bladder and urinary problems are common after hysterectomy. One of the reasons for this is that when the uterus is in its natural position it provides support to the bladder. When the uterus is removed, some of that support is compromised.

Bowel problems are also common. Without its natural support, the bowel moves down and takes up the space where the uterus had been. Without the uterus separating the bowel from the bladder, when there is stool in the bowel it creates pressure on the bladder by pressing directly against it. The bowel bulges down creating a rectocele, which is a ballooning of the bowel into the vagina.

When the nerves that attach to the uterus are severed, sensation in the vagina, clitoris, labia, and nipples is diminished or lost entirely.

Many women develop a permanent searing pain of the nerve pathways that radiate down from the waist through the buttock to the back of the knee, making it painful to sit or walk. Some women experience what they describe as cyclical electric shocks in the vagina as a result of damage to the pelvic nerves. This makes it difficult to sit and often interferes with sleep and other normal activities.

Physical sexual sensation is diminished or lost entirely because of the severing of nerves and the removal of the uterus. Women who experienced uterine orgasm before the surgery will not experience it after the surgery, because the uterine contractions that occur during uterine orgasm cannot occur without a uterus.

The loss of uterine orgasm will only be missed by women who experienced it before the surgery. Although a small number of hysterectomized women experience slight vaginal wall contractions, most women report a total loss of sexual feeling.

Severing the blood supply to the uterus diminishes the blood flow in the pelvis and to the external genitalia, including the ovaries, vagina, labia, and clitoris, as well as the legs and feet.

One of the many functions of the uterus and the ovaries is cardiovascular protection. When the uterus is removed, women have a three-times greater incidence of heart disease. When the ovaries are removed, women have a seven-times greater incidence of heart disease.

A woman's ovaries—her gonads—continue to produce hormones her entire lifetime. Oophorectomy (the surgical removal of the ovaries) is performed on about 75% of the women who undergo hysterectomy. The medically correct term for the removal of the gonads is castration.

Because of damage to the blood supply to the ovaries, there is a loss of ovarian function in 35-40% of the women whose ovaries are not removed during hysterectomy. This too results in a loss of ovarian function, which is the same as castration.

During a vaginal hysterectomy the uterus is removed through the vagina. Because the uterus is continuous with the cervix which is continuous with the vagina, the surgeon cuts into the vagina around the cervix, creating a hole in the top of the vagina. This hole must then be sutured shut, forming a closed pocket and a shortened vagina.

Because the cervix is no longer there, the top of the vagina is sutured to one or more of the severed ligaments. Because the suture sometimes does not hold, hysterectomized women commonly report prolapse of the vagina out of the vaginal opening, much like a pocket that is turned inside out.

During an abdominal hysterectomy, a horizontal incision is made across the pelvis above the pubic bone. Depending on the size of the uterus, it is then either pulled out through the vagina or through the pelvic incision.

Total abdominal hysterectomy (TAH) and total vaginal hysterectomy (TVH) is the removal of the uterus and the cervix. Partial hysterectomy is the removal of the body of the uterus, leaving the cervical stump.

A laparoscopic-assisted vaginal hysterectomy (LAVH) involves inflating the abdomen and pelvis with gas/air and removing the uterus either vaginally or by cutting it into small pieces that are pulled out through the navel (the belly button). This type of hysterectomy requires a minimum of three small incisions. It takes longer to perform than other types of hysterectomy, so there is an increased risk of complications from anesthesia, perforation of the bladder and bowel, and stress on all of the internal organs (including the heart) as a result of the pressure created by inflating the abdomen.

Whether TAH, TVH, or LAVH, the vagina is surgically shortened and made into a closed pocket, because the hole at the top of the vagina must be sutured shut.

No matter how good the surgeon's skill or technique, and no matter what type of hysterectomy is performed, the result is the same: a hormone-responsive reproductive sex organ is removed.

The physical changes are far-reaching. The most consistent problems women experience after hysterectomy are a loss of sexual feeling, a loss of vitality, joint pain, profound fatigue, and personality change.

The internal female genital organs have lifelong functions that can never be replaced. There is never an age or a time in a woman's life when her uterus and ovaries are not essential to her health and wellbeing.[103]

When I was done Rick was surprised that it took me only about 10 minutes. So he asked me repeat it, he typed it up, and now it's the standard brief anatomy lesson at HERS, which we call "Female Anatomy: the Functions of the Female Organs." It's the minimum information women require to understand their bodies and to make informed decisions about medical choices. It should be made available on every hospital, doctor, and government health website.

---

[103] http://hersfoundation.org/anatomy/index.html.

THIRTY-TWO

"Fruscration—frustrated, fractured, lost."

Camden, New Jersey—Rick Schweikert

The daughter of a protestor named Alice drove her mother quite a distance to join us in New Jersey. She sat down beside the Cooper University Hospital sign, watching her mother protest. A few minutes later I overheard her saying she was leaving and would return to give Alice a ride home.

"I don't think she approves of her mom protesting," I said to Nora.

"I don't know," Nora replied, "this might be a case where there's more than meets the eye."

After undergoing a hysterectomy, Alice's mom seemed to be doing okay for a few months. But then she crashed. And then she was in such a bad way she stopped getting out of bed. Her family didn't understand what was going on, but her daughter couldn't stand to watch her mom suffer. She searched for information that could help Alice, but all she found was the same thing over and over again...how women are better than ever after the surgery. Finally, she found HERS.

"Alice would barely eat or talk," Nora said. "When her daughter got me on the phone I told her to put the receiver to her mom's ear. Her mom listened, then cried softly for a long time, but then she finally began to speak to me. She didn't say much. She mostly just listened while I told her that I understood what she was experiencing."

Many of the women who call HERS go through a similar process. "Typically," Nora said, "a couple of weeks after the surgery there's a short lived kind of euphoria, an adrenalin rush." Nora thinks this phase is the body's way of trying to rise to the challenge of coping with the devastating shock of sudden, dramatic changes. But that euphoria soon dissipates, and then comes the crash. "It's not a true depression," Nora said, "it's more of a melancholy, a deep sadness and overwhelming awareness of loss, nearly incomprehensible to anyone who hasn't experienced it. It's intensely painful, and more physical than emotional."

Alice now knew the pain and loss were permanent, and that validation was what she needed to be able to cope a little better. She was grateful to her daughter, because she never would've found HERS otherwise.

Two police officers pulled up from opposite directions, talking to each other through their driver's-side windows. After they drove on, one of them circled the block and waved us over to her window. "Can I have one of those?" she asked. Nora gave her a pamphlet, and a few more to hand out back at the precinct. "Thank you. Here's my card. Give me a call if you have any trouble. It's great what you're doing."

A protestor named Donna lived within walking distance of the hospital. A doctor told her she needed a hysterectomy because she had large fibroids. Even if they could be removed, the doctor said, more fibroids would grow back in their place. The doctor's advice was nonsense, because she was beyond the age when new fibroids tend to develop.

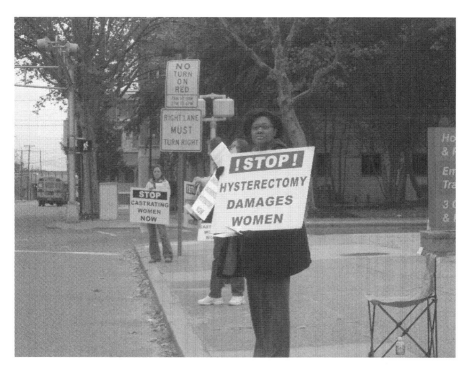

Nora helped Donna find a doctor who had the ability to perform a myomectomy and successfully remove the fibroids. Any lingering doubts about her decision vanished after she attended her first protest and spoke to other women.

One of the women who wasn't so fortunate was a protestor named Charlene. After the surgery, along with the rest of the most common adverse effects, Charlene suffered from neuropathy, and her feet throbbed with pain if they got either hot or cold. It was a chilly day, and it was obvious Charlene was struggling to be out there. Because she wasn't able to stand on her feet very long, she brought a folding chair with her to the Camden protest. But her need to warn other women and her need to express the anger she felt was more important than being comfortable. I thought about Charlene a lot after the Camden protest.

In the same way that the seven seas aren't really so much a series of isolated oceans as they are one global river flowing around the seven continents, so too our body isn't so much a collection of isolated organs as it is one interconnected whole. Every part of a woman's body is altered by the removal of the female organs. Charlene knew that attending the protest wouldn't improve the problems she was experiencing, but it would give her peace of mind that she was out there telling doctors and hospital administrators how angry she was.

Sarah, Sharon, and a few others also joined us. We distributed several boxes of pamphlets. And in Camden we saw it all, as they say. A few nurses nearly spit at us they were so angry we were out there, but others were supportive. One nurse even hugged me.

There was a street vendor near the hospital. Not long after the nurse hugged me, another group of nurses were on break getting a snack. When we tried giving them pamphlets they laughed at us. A little while later one of those same nurses walked by and was irritated to be offered a pamphlet a second time, but she took it. The third time she took another pamphlet and asked a few brisk questions. Each time after that, she said hello and asked how we were doing. Before long she was asking us questions, telling us about her job, convincing her coworkers to read the pamphlet.

On the other end of the spectrum, a female gynecologist stormed through our protest, saying, "Hysterectomy is good for women, it doesn't damage them!" She marched away from us with her arms pumping back and forth, her shoes pounding the pavement on the way to the parking lot. A minute later she screeched around the corner in her fancy sports car.

One woman I talked with in Camden said, "Not all women are unhappy with their hysterectomies." All I said to her was, "What was your life like before your surgery," and she froze. Her eyes seemed to glaze over, and finally she said, "I know you're right. I can't do half the things I did before the surgery. I was just hoping one day I'd wake up and I'd be my old self again. But that's never going to happen, is it?" Then she slowly walked away.

About 2.5 million people visit the HERS website each year. The following email is from a woman living near Camden who spent years searching for validation for the problems hysterectomy caused her:

> I DO NOT KNOW HOW I FOUND THIS WEB SITE..BUT AM SO THANKFUL I DID...2001 HAD HYSTER.WITH OVARIES REMOVED.. ALSO PROLAPSE (SEVERE) REPAIR...2001 WAS THE LAST TIME I HAD SEX...NEVER WAS TOLD, NEVER TOLD ANYONE,WAS LOST AND FELT SO ALONE UNTIL I FOUND THIS PAGE. I AM 60 AND HAD 4 CHILDREN... ALWAYS HAD AN ACTIVE SEX LIFE AND THEN —GONE....AND SO ALONE...FELT IT WAS ME....TODAY I WENT TO MY THERA-PIST (WOMaN AGE 40+) TOLD HER ABOUT THIS AND SHE SAYS HER CLIENTS HAVE SAID THE SAME THING...SHE SAID MEN ARE ALWAYS TOLD OF ANY POSSIBLE AD-VERSE AFFECTS...WHAT CAN I DO? I HAVE 2 DAUGHTERS AND WOULD ALWAYS ADVISE AGAINST THIS. THANKS FOR BEING OUT THERE

Women often tell me hysterectomy is a good thing, until they find out I'm the author of *un becoming* and they realize it's safe to talk with me. Then they take a step closer, their voices change, and the floodgates open. They tell me all the problems they're having, and I suggest they call HERS.

Many of the hysterectomized women I meet take anti-depressants and say, "I thought I was losing my mind until I found HERS." They have no one to validate their experiences and begin to question their sanity. When they're suddenly confronted with someone who understands, the relief is tremendous.

HERS offers no placebos, no happy pills, no sugar-coated messages. Only information as it's reported by hundreds of thousands of women and a century of medical literature. Most women who call HERS cancel the surgery, or wish they'd known about HERS before it was too late.

One guy told me his mom walked to Cooper for a checkup before her hysterectomy the afternoon after our first day there. She spotted one of the pamphlets on the ground with a shoeprint on it. She picked it up, he said, and he was stopping by to tell us she canceled the surgery and wanted a clean pamphlet for herself and the doctor. I asked him how many he wanted, and he said, "Just two. I'd hate to waste them."

Around noon, a Harley Davidson motorcycle pulled up in a no parking zone. And then a few more pulled up on the sidewalk. Before we knew it, there were about 50 of them, and by the time we stopped protesting, there were maybe a 100 bikes parked in rows in front of the hospital. It was some kind of toys-for-kids drive the bikers were organizing. One of the lasting images from the Protest & Play year was one of those bearded bikers reclining on his Harley, soaking up the sun as he read a HERS pamphlet.

A woman came out of the medical building across the street. "I'm gonna have one of those," she said. Nora asked her why, and she shrugged her shoulders, saying, "Because they said I need it, and it don't cost me nothin. Maybe I got a prolapse or something, I don't know." Nora asked for her address so she could send her some materials, but the woman said she was homeless. She walked away reading her pamphlet, saying she'd call Nora if she could get to a phone. We never thought we'd hear from her again, but she came to the protest the next day. After speaking with Nora a while longer about using a pessary and exercises to resolve her mild prolapse, she said she was canceling the surgery.

Preserving Medicaid for the needy may be as easy as preventing fraudulent doctors from appropriating taxpayer dollars for unnecessary surgeries.

The doctor had apparently neglected to mention to her that exercises and a pessary would most likely relieve the symptoms caused by her prolapsed uterus. Prolapse of the uterus is fairly common, particularly in women who've had several children, had labor induced or accelerated, or had difficult vaginal deliveries where a doctor pulled the baby out of the vagina.

There are three degrees of uterine prolapse. Most women are unaware of a first-degree prolapse, unless a doctor mentions it during a pelvic exam, because the first degree is slight and without symptoms. With a second-degree prolapse the uterus has descended a little more, and the cervix may be at the opening of the vagina. In a third-degree prolapse, the cervix and sometimes the uterus protrude outside of the vaginal opening. Women with a third-degree prolapse often worry that the uterus will actually drop out onto the floor. Although stretched, the ligaments in the pelvis remain attached to the uterus, so it's not possible for the uterus to fall out of the body.

The most common treatment options are, from the least to most invasive, exercises (to strengthen the muscles of the vagina and abdomen to better support the uterus), pessary (a rubber, plastic, or metal ring in which the cervix rests, designed to support the uterus and correct the prolapse), and uterine suspension (suturing the uterus to other tissue for support).

Doctors sometimes recommend Kegel exercises. They may help somewhat, but there's a modification of the Kegel exercises that seems to give more significant if not total resolution of a first or second degree prolapse: Sitting down (the best vaginal muscle control is achieved when sitting), tighten the vaginal and abdominal muscles, and then quickly release them. Repeat ten times. Then tighten the vaginal and abdominal muscles and hold for the count of ten, then release. Repeat ten times. It's essential that these exercises be performed three times a day, every day, to know for sure if you're seeing improvement. You'll know within two months if the exercises are resolving your prolapse. If you don't experience significant improvement within two months of doing the exercises three times a day, then they aren't going to work for you. If you do experience significant improvement, you'll need to continue the exercises on a daily basis.

Lifting that causes a pulling sensation in the pelvis will worsen a prolapse. One way to alleviate the stress on the pelvis is to hold objects close to your body while lifting them, rather than having your arms outstretched away from your body. If you can't hug the object close to your body when lifting it, then it's best not to.

A prolapsed uterus may also pull the bladder (cystocele) and part of the bowel (rectocele) down into the vagina. In a slight (first degree), moderate (second degree), and sometimes in a severe (third degree) prolapse, a pessary is frequently all that's needed for support and to relieve incontinence. Pessaries come in many different shapes and sizes. Some doctors don't keep a large inventory on hand, but it's important to find one that works for you.

As it progresses from second to third degree, the prolapse may cause lower back pain, a pulling sensation in the lower pelvis, and vaginal pressure. In that case, if the pessary doesn't work, you might consider surgical resuspension of the uterus and repair of the cystocele. During a uterine resuspension, a horizontal incision is made above the pubic bone. The surgeon then shortens the stretched ligaments with sutures, and the uterus is sutured to soft tissue in the pelvis. It's still a major surgery, but it's far less invasive than hysterectomy, and you'll retain the functions of your female organs.

The New Jersey reading of *un becoming* was held at the Princeton Center for Yoga and Health. The reading in Philadelphia the next week had already been organized, so I asked The Brick Playhouse if they'd be willing to drive up to Princeton to present a reading of the play there too. They agreed, so the same cast was scheduled to do back-to-back readings in Princeton and Philadelphia.

One of the actors happened to be a nurse, which was always a hit-or-miss situation. About half of the actors throughout the year who worked in the medical industry were supportive, the other half weren't. This nurse wasn't in the least supportive, and there wasn't a lot I could do about it once I arrived. The first email I got from her was dismissive and loaded with the usual myths about hysterectomy. She believed what she had been taught and wasn't interested in the facts. I mailed her a stack of medical journal articles, but I never got a response.

Though we didn't see eye to eye, her negativity and cynicism contributed nicely to her portrayal of Dr. Rose Parker, an arrogant female gynecologist character in the play. And the direction by Bill McKinlay of The Brick Playhouse was excellent.

One couple in the audience from Japan took pamphlets with them to send back to friends in Tokyo, where they said hysterectomy was becoming a big problem.

Nora's friend Isabel—an above-the-knee amputee since childhood—also attended the reading. She said, "Hysterectomy is a major handicap. People say I'm handicapped, but in many ways I'm more whole with the loss of a limb than a woman is without her uterus."

THIRTY-THREE

What women tell women.

Philadelphia, Pennsylvania—Rick Schweikert

I asked a board member of a rural Pennsylvania hospital what he knew about hysterectomy rates at their hospital. He didn't know, but he said the hospital was recently forced to defend itself from a spate of malpractice lawsuits. "So the board voted to order a Tissue Committee to randomly review some of our hysterectomies," he said, "and a lot of the reports came back negative."

"Negative meaning the surgeries were unnecessary?"

"That's right. And then, because of the oversight, the number of hysterectomies being performed starting going down. A fraction of what they were doing before."

"Really? Well that's telling," I said. "Is the Tissue Committee still doing oversight?"

"No. It's pretty expensive paying someone to review all those pathology reports. And the doctors made a plea to the board."

"To let them go back to performing unnecessary surgeries?"

"They didn't exactly put it that way. They convinced enough board members that hysterectomies were elective and women want them, even if we had to defend ourselves from a few lawsuits here and there. They also said if they weren't allowed to perform them at our hospital, they'd do them elsewhere."

"With your competition."

"A few of us voted to keep a close eye on the doctors, but we were outvoted after a financial review said revenue was declining. The board recommended encouraging them to use more caution in prescribing surgeries and to review their own pathology reports."

"In other words, they were told to monitor themselves. Then what happened?"

"The number of hysterectomies went back up again."

"And revenue too."

"That's right. The overall expense of defending the hospital from lawsuits was minor compared to the revenue the operating rooms were bringing in."

I called Nora to tell her about the conversation, and she was disgusted by it, but not surprised. "The complicity of the hospital board," Nora said, "is similar to Ford Motor Company's decision to continue making Pinto cars in the 1970s after they knew Pintos exploded upon rear impact.[104] It cost them less money to compensate the families of the people killed and injured in those accidents than it would've cost them in lost revenue, so they continued selling lethal cars until Ralph Nader blew the whistle on them. Even then, the government quailed to Ford's lobbyists and delayed taking action to protect the public. In both instances," Nora said, "lives were expendable in the name of profit."

The amazing Joan was with us again in Philly, as were Debbie, Ernie, Ted, Marlis, Jim, and others. In the cool late-morning shadow of the hospital, I tore open the first box of materials and handed a stack to Joan. Before I could do the same for the next protestor, I heard a doctor say, "Hysterectomies are elective! Why are you protesting against this hospital?"

Joan replied, "Not one of the women protesting here knew what her life would be like after the surgery."

---

[104] Dowie, Mark, "Pinto Madness," *Mother Jones*, September 1977.

The doctor snatched the pamphlet from her and shoved it into the pocket of his white coat.

A few days before the protest, Nora and I papered the hospital with HERS pamphlets. Along the way, she asked a few people where we could find the office of Robert Giuntoli, the doctor who hysterectomized and castrated her. Someone sitting at a desk in a filthy, dilapidated office said, "No, there's no Dr. Giuntoli here. Oh, wait a minute….Didn't he die? I don't know."

As we walked away, Nora told me that when she was finally able to walk again after the surgery, she searched for a specialist who could help her understand how she could've been so healthy and vibrant before the surgery, and suddenly so debilitated afterwards. When she couldn't find any answers, she went to the medical library at Penn and did her own research.

Every day for two years she researched journal articles and medical textbooks. It wasn't long before she began to more fully understand female anatomy and why sex organs are so important to health and wellbeing. She also found medical journal articles going back a hundred years attesting to the fact that hysterectomy is damaging and should never be done except in life-or-death situations. Then Nora paid a visit to Giuntoli's office to tell him what she learned.

She told Giuntoli in detail how his actions had damaged her body and ruined her life. When he attempted to interrupt her, she told him, "Sit down and be quiet. I didn't come here to listen to you. I came here to tell you that I now understand what you did to me." She told Giuntoli how he'd damaged her body, her sex life, her health, and her family. A few weeks later Nora heard that Giuntoli had a massive coronary. She said, "It may not be the nicest thing to say, but it was minutely satisfying knowing that for the rest of his life he'd worry about having another heart attack every time he had sex."

On October 6, 1983, Nora and Giuntoli were interviewed by Lindacarol Graham in the Philadelphia Daily News. The middle of the page was dominated by the female symbol ♀, which took up more print area than the text of the interviews. Giuntoli's interview was to the right of the symbol. Nora's interview was to the left. Graham never mentions that Giuntoli was the doctor who hysterectomized Nora, and there are a number of errors and omissions of fact.

That was Nora's first interview. It taught her what questions to ask before she agreed to an interview. Now when a reporter approaches her, she asks them, "What made you interested in this subject?" and "Whose press release did you receive?" Those two questions reveal if the journalist's slant is likely to promote a doctor's practice or promoting a new drug or medical device, which is the motivation behind many health articles.

Nora was especially fearless about getting arrested here, eager for the press it would've generated. She trespassed onto hospital property, carrying a sign and distributing pamphlets at the main entrance. But the hospital did nothing. They apparently didn't want to draw anymore attention to the protest.

There were a lot of parents who were visiting their children at the university. One girl took a pamphlet from us, held it close to her chest, and walked down the street that way, lagging behind her father who scolded her to catch up. Her mother slipped quickly down the block ahead of them, averting her eyes from our signs. When her daughter caught up with her, her mother snatched the pamphlet from her and threw it into the garbage.

Another family was hurried through our protest by their embarrassed father. "Come on, come on!" he yelled to his college-aged daughter. But his wife said, "John, just relax, will you?" His wife took a pamphlet from us, telling her daughter, "Go ahead, take one." Her daughter then asked, "What's a hysterectomy?" Her father walked ahead of them as her mother put her arm around her daughter's shoulder, talking with her as they continued down the street.

One female gynecologist wouldn't take a pamphlet, so Nora said, "It's information I'm sure would be helpful to you." The doctor replied, "No, no, no!" as she snatched the pamphlet out of Nora's hand and stuffed it into her pocket, hurrying toward the main entrance.

Nora tried to hand a pamphlet to another young doctor who said, "No thanks. I'm a chiropractor."

"Do you help your patients make a connection between hysterectomy and back pain?" Nora asked.

The doctor stopped and pondered the question. "No," he said, "I guess I never thought about it."

"When the uterine ligaments are severed, it destroys the structural integrity of the pelvis, the hips widen, and the spine compresses. Of course you know that one of those ligaments is the utero-sacral ligament, which attaches to the uterus and the sacrum in the lower back. There are more than 22 million women alive today who've been hysterectomized, and the majority of them experience back pain after the surgery. But you've never made the connection?"

"No, but maybe I'll start asking them," the doctor said.

"A lot of chiropractors ask women if they've had a hysterectomy right on the questionnaire they're given before their first appointment," Nora said.

"Not a bad idea," he said. "Thanks," and he walked away.

My usual icebreaker with a doctor was something like, "Here's some information you should be aware of," or, "Here's some helpful information for your clients." Most of the responses I got at Penn were either completely preposterous or very rude, like the doctor who said, "The female uterus is a delicacy in some parts of South America," laughing as he walked away. Others said, "Oh, just f___ off."

One doctor said with a big smile, "We don't do unnecessary hysterectomies."

"That's not true," I said, "HERS has counseled hundreds of women who were operated on at Penn."

"Well, we don't," he said.

"These women right here protesting with me were hysterectomized here—"

But before I could finish my sentence he flippantly said again, "Nope, we don't," and he was gone.

The Philly reading of *un becoming* was held at the Community Education Center, on Lancaster Avenue. Usually the cast would stick around for the talkback that followed the reading, but the Brick Playhouse cast quickly filed out of the theater and was gone, which was unfortunate because they missed really good talkbacks in both cities.

Many years earlier, before Nora was hysterectomized, she had asked her friend Teresa whether she had any sexual changes from the surgery. Teresa told Nora sex was better than ever and the hysterectomy was the best thing she ever did. After the surgery, Nora told Teresa that she had no sexual feeling and asked Teresa why she said sex was better than ever. Teresa's response was, "Oh,

I didn't want to worry you." Until then, Nora had wondered why Teresa and her husband slept in separate bedrooms.

Nora went on to found HERS, and she was thrust into the media spotlight. About five years later, Nora was interviewed on a major television talk show. Teresa's mother saw the show, and when she was in town visiting from Florida she told Teresa's mother told her to ask Nora if they could come over for a visit. "That's what's wrong with my legs and my back...and my arms too," Teresa's mother said when they arrived at Nora's. She hadn't associated the problems she was experiencing with the surgery until she saw Nora on TV. The result is that hysterectomy became her daughter's legacy, which her daughter helped to perpetuate by passing it on to Nora.

Now, all these years later, Teresa attended the Philly reading of *un becoming* with her husband Philip. After the play they quietly thanked me. It was one of the many times that year when I felt like no matter how much I learn about hysterectomy, I'll never fully understand why more women aren't screaming in the streets about what's being done.

An email we recently received from a woman in Pittsburgh provides a glimpse into why another family wasn't able to help each other and why gynecologists can't really be trusted:

> I am so angry because of my ignorance and lack of a second opinion, lack of reading the info that HERS Foundation had given me prior to my surgery but refused to hear anyone but the doctor whom I recently see in a different light. I feel so misinformed, so cheated and know how my life is so different just by watching my sisters and mother go thru the same changes as a result of there recent hysterectomies. Sometimes

it is "hard to see the picture when you are in the frame" but now i realize how my body looks, feel and the compared symptoms that we face everyday. This is the worst thing that has every happened to us. We identify with at least 90% of the facts. This is definitely contrary to what I discussed with my ex-gynecologist.

It was always satisfying when someone in the audience would personally relate to one of the characters. In Philly an artist named Tess saw herself in the character Emma Douglas. She avoided a hysterectomy after being counseled by Nora, and she said the similarities between her life and Emma's were remarkable.

It's fitting to conclude the Pennsylvania chapter with another journal entry from Joan:

The University of Pennsylvania Hospital was an incredibly busy place, more so than NYC even, and I stayed an extra day. We handed out huge amounts of materials. One of the protesters, Marlis (who's husband Jim joined us), had her hysterectomy performed by a female gynecologist at the University of Pennsylvania in January 2004. She was terribly damaged by it, both physically and mentally, and wanted to sue. When she complained about the adverse effects, her doctor was rude to her. Another volunteer, an executive at American Airlines who avoided a hysterectomy because of HERS, flew in from Dallas for the weekend to participate in the protest. There were lots of medical people walking around—some accepted the pamphlets and some would not. One young female medical student was quite interested in what we had to say since it provided her with a patient's viewpoint. Another female hospital employee said that she would come back the next day to help us distribute our materials because she would be off work and felt so strongly about our cause. She showed up the following morning and assisted us for an hour. It was appreciated as we welcomed all the help we could get.

The day I was to fly back to Michigan the concierge of the Inn at Penn Hotel, a woman in her early 40's, disclosed that her gynecologist had been trying to persuade her for a few years to have a hysterectomy because she was having heavy bleeding. She really didn't want to have it. I told her briefly about the adverse effects and she gladly accepted the pamphlets and was so thankful to me. I was later informed that she had contacted the HERS Foundation and advised them that she would definitely not have the surgery after reviewing the educational brochures.

The New Jersey and Pennsylvania protests were two of the most memorable ones of the year. It was nice spending time with Nora again in her home, something we hadn't been able to do since the protest year began. It also gave Nora a much-needed two-week break from having to get on a plane.

THIRTY-FOUR

If the female organs hung outside a woman's body, sexual

function would be apparent.

Wilmington, Delaware—Nora W. Coffey

It was only a short time ago that women won the right to vote, own property, and were provided with legal protection from rape by their husbands. Each right was hard-fought. Full knowledge about the aftermath of hysterectomy and castration is another right we'll have to fight hard for. But make no mistake about it, we will win this battle.

For now, most women don't have any way of knowing that the uterus and ovaries are as important to health and wellbeing as the penis and testicles are so very important to men.

There's an absurd amount of misinformation out there about gender biology. For nearly half a century, women and men who've wanted to change their sex have been led to believe that all they had to do was have their sex organs removed and take synthetic hormones. But although the operation may help a person become a transvestite and gender-identify with the opposite sex (or, more importantly for some, to un-gender identify with the sex they were born with), no doctor can change a Y chromosome to an X chromosome. This notion has been advanced by the media in articles like the November 21, 1966 *New York Times* news report that said, "The Johns Hopkins Hospital has quietly begun performing sex change surgery." As well as in movies like *Dog Day Afternoon*, in which a trio of gunmen rob a bank in order to raise money for a "sex change operation." At the end of the movie the character

Leon has the operation and becomes a woman. Although you will be "changed" by the removal of your sex organs, changing sexes is biologically impossible. In such an environment of misinformation, how is anyone to know who to believe?

I was joined at the Christiana Health System Hospital in Wilmington by a single mother who was never married. And because she was single, her pregnancy, she said, was treated like a contagious disease. She felt doctors pushed her toward a hysterectomy because having a baby out of marriage was unacceptable in the doctor's judgment. "It was like I didn't deserve to have a uterus if I was going to use it this way," she said. She avoided surgery, though, after finding HERS.

Her situation rang true with me. Many women I counsel feel that hysterectomy is a judgment against them for a number of reasons: being overweight, poor, lesbian, black, not physically attractive, or simply smarter or more confident than the doctor. It's a powerful position for a doctor to be in, to exact such a judgment against women for living lives the doctors envy, find threatening, or deem unacceptable.

I've often wondered if some doctors feel that by taking these powerful organs from strong women their power will somehow accrue to them, become part of them, and make them stronger, smarter, sexier. Doctors are in a unique capacity to wield this power, and they do it legally. In fact, they're handsomely compensated for it and shielded from criminal prosecution.

At some point I caught wind of a very strong odor coming from a nearby bus stop shelter. I found a homeless woman inside who clearly hadn't bathed in a very long time. When we made eye contact, she looked shell-shocked, like a war refugee.

She was barely recognizable as a human. She wore filthy rags, and the odor was so intense it was difficult getting near her. I gave her a pamphlet, and she attempted to speak. Her speech was so garbled I couldn't understand what she was saying. She looked down at the pamphlet and then back up at me. I smiled, and finally the muscles of her cracked face slowly softened. As I walked away she was still smiling at me.

More than 78% of hysterectomized women report a change in personality. More than 77% report a "loss of energy" and "profound fatigue." More than 66% report "short term memory loss." More than 64% say they're "unable to maintain home" and more than 48% say they're "unable to maintain previous level of employment." More than 58% of hysterectomized women report "insomnia" and 68% report "difficulty relating with and interacting with others."[105] When a woman becomes permanently disabled, her friends and family may console her and support her for a while, but her family will soon need to go on with their lives, even if her problems won't go away.

For many women a steady income is the difference between needing public assistance—if she can get it—or being independent. Her predicament then becomes about a lot more than money. Losing her independence can make a woman feel like a failure. This can spill over into other parts of her life. More than 75% of hysterectomized women report a "diminished or absent sexual desire." Her disabilities and the loss of income contribute to strained relationships, as does the physiologic loss of sexuality and sexual feeling.

---

[105] "Adverse Effects Data," HERS Foundation, www.hersfoundation.org/effects.html.

On average, the women counseled by HERS seek the help of 25 doctors within the first year after surgery. Those doctors inflict more and more damage with experimental drugs and treatments. And more surgeries. Women who need to believe that a remedy exists find themselves in a conundrum of spending money they don't have to seek a cure that doesn't exist. One problem leads to the next. She may not have family to help out in hard times. She may have no choice but to get food stamps to feed her children. She may not be able to cover the rent or the mortgage.

Many women have called HERS from homeless shelters, domestic abuse centers, and prisons. Some of the women who have called HERS from prison had no criminal history prior to the hysterectomy.

I counseled a woman named Rowena Leonard who was a construction project manager. She was strong, she liked hard work, and she never got sick. She had no medical problems at all, but her gynecologist convinced her she needed a hysterectomy for fibroids. Her first day back to work after the surgery she got into her pickup as usual and worked a full day. But she doesn't remember any of it. A few days later she was in a state prison. At some point she got into a car, drove to Chicago, and held up a bank at gunpoint.

She had no idea how she acquired a gun, and she didn't need the money. When she left the bank, witnesses say she strolled out onto the street as if she'd done nothing wrong. She seemed surprised to suddenly find herself surrounded by police. She said it wasn't until the media shined their lights on her that she realized she had a gun in her hand. She then put the gun to her head and pulled the trigger. The bullet is still lodged there.

She asked me to testify in court on her behalf. Her counsel mounted a defense that was parallel to *non compos mentis* cases of postpartum depression. Her attorney found highly respected experts who testified about hormone shock when the ovaries are removed. Before the trial, Rowena's lawyer told me he was assured by the judge he wouldn't send her to prison. Rowena expected to get probation and community service and go home in her white suit. Instead, the judge found her guilty, and Rowena was handcuffed and taken to Cook County prison.

In Wilmington, a very dapper man said, "My wife had that a long time ago. She went down hill real quick after that one." He stood there reading the pamphlet cover to cover, noting all the health problems his wife had over the years. "One day she went in for a check up, and now she never leaves the house." He spoke of her hysterectomy as a tragic accident, but it was no accident.

THIRTY-FIVE

The priorities of a nation.

Morgantown, West Virginia—Rick Schweikert

Violence is the most prevalent and immediate problem facing American women today. And aside from murder, hysterectomy is the ultimate violence against women. What other problem would elicit the thousands upon thousands of emails HERS receives year after year from all corners of the globe like the one below:

> I just read the list of "symptoms" [on the HERS website] found after a hysterectomy with removal of ovaries. I was "terminated" by the surgeon (jerk) who did my surgery because I told him I was having MAJOR difficulties and he laughed at me and told me I needed to see a shrink. I attempted suicide 3 months after my surgery and checked myself into a "psych" hospital a year afterwards because I was VERY irritable and angry all the time. I was diagnosed as Bipolar, yet I do not believe the diagnosis as I didn't have problems until this terrible surgery... I no longer want to have sex, no longer speak to friends and have not been able to hold a job since that day in September 2005 when they "castrated" me... WHAT CAN I DO TO HELP GET THE WORD OUT so nobody has to go through what I have gone through the past year?

It's a side of human nature that's difficult to look in the eye. Gynecologists sanction, perpetrate, and then deny any wrongdoing as they cause others to suffer—the very thing they swore to prevent. It's harder still to accept that their colleagues in other branches of medicine are complicit.

As Albert Einstein said, "The world is a dangerous place, not because of those who do evil, but because of those who look on and do nothing."

Every day, more than 1,700 women needlessly undergo this senseless brutality, and every day three of those women will die before leaving the hospital. In his article titled "Why Aren't We Shocked?" Bob Herbert writes:

> The relentless violence against women and girls is linked at its core to the wider society's casual willingness to dehumanize women and girls, to see them first and foremost as sexual vessels—objects—and never, ever as the equals of men... "Once you dehumanize somebody, everything is possible," said Taina Bien-Aimé, executive director of the women's advocacy group Equality Now.[106]

I asked Sutapa Basu, executive director of the Women's Center at the University of Washington in Seattle, what she thought was the biggest problem facing American women. "Violence," she said. "In all its forms. From rape on campus to modern-day slavery, another woman is abused in this country every nine seconds." That statistic doesn't include surgical violence.

Episode 8 of the second season of the TV show *Grey's Anatomy* is a poignant example of the subtleties of institutionalized violence against women. A woman doctor performs a hysterectomy, castration, and double mastectomy on one of her best friends. The catch is, her friend doesn't have a medical problem. She's afraid she might die because a family member died of cancer, but she doesn't have cancer. Another doctor hovering around the scene is confused why the surgeon is willing to perform the operation,

---

[106] Herbert, Bob, "Why Aren't We Shocked?" *New York Times*, October 16, 2006.

making the point that if a man's sex organs were hanging in the balance the story would be different. Not only does the female surgeon proceed with the unwarranted surgery, she tells her husband (also a surgeon) to mind his own business when he speaks up for their mutual friend who she's about to operate on.[107]

Many of the women who contact HERS are resigned to the surgery and only make the call to get basic post-operative information—when they'll be able to drive a car, take a bath, or have sex. But when they discover what the doctor isn't telling them, they often cancel the surgery. When informed consent is present, women almost never go ahead with the surgery.

In Morgantown there was no public space for us to stage our protest in front of the Ruby Memorial Medical Center, a teaching hospital affiliated with West Virginia University (WVU). There was a Mountaineers home football game that weekend, and the university was besieged by football fans. When we drove up the long hospital driveway, a police officer stopped us. "If you don't have a written appointment with a doctor, you can't get through," he said.

"What if we had an emergency?" I asked.

The officer shrugged his shoulders and waved us away, so we had no way of knowing if other protestors showed up in Morgantown.

We parked elsewhere and walked back to paper cars in the hospital parking lot and other lots around town. We also went inside the hospital and left pamphlets everywhere we could.

---

[107] Rhimes, Shonda and Schmir, Mimi, "Let It Be," *Grey's Anatomy*, Season 2, Episode 8, November13, 2005.

None of the women's groups at WVU responded to our emails, phone calls, or letters. Because we got no response from the WVU Women's Studies faculty, we were surprised six months later when a student group from WVU invited us back to campus.

Members of a group called the Female Equality Movement (FEM) asked us during a women's studies conference in Maryland if we'd bring *un becoming* to WVU a few months after our Protest & Play year would end. With that second visit to Morgantown, we made an extra effort to get in touch with media and to make arrangements for Nora to speak to women's studies classes. She got invited to speak to a handful of students in a very small, poorly attended classroom, and the reading itself was sparsely attended, even by FEM members. The group's website says the biggest problems facing women today are "pay inequity, reproductive freedom, sexual assault, voter registration and political participation, body image, health issues, stereotyping and discrimination."

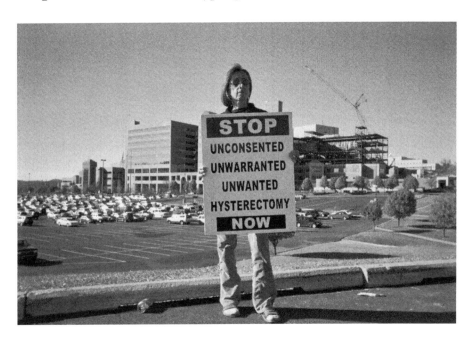

Whether we're talking to Women's Studies departments, Women's Centers, community groups, or yoga instructors, the way hysterectomy is perceived varies greatly. They each have different issues, so they each have different concerns. But when we hear testimony from a woman in Africa whose clitoris was amputated, many of us respond with fear, anger, empathy, and sadness. So why don't we respond the same way when the sex organs of American women are amputated?

THIRTY-SIX

"Every woman in my church."

Kansas City, Kansas—Rick Schweikert

The construction site at the Kansas University Medical Center was like no other hospital expansion we'd see that year. The main intersection at the corner of the sprawling medical campus was boarded up with signs that read, "Danger!" and "KEEP OUT!" while funneling customers inside.

As this book demonstrates, America's hospitals and clinics need consumer warning labels at every entrance, alerting the public about hospital-borne infections, medical errors, negligence, and medically unwarranted surgeries.

Almost two million people catch potentially fatal infections upon entering America's hospitals. Methicillin-resistant staphylococcus aureus (MRSA), an antibiotic-resistant "superbug" that can survive on cloth and plastic for up to 90 days, accounts for 59% of those infections. One in every 20 hospital patients carries MRSA.[108] The chairman of the Committee to Reduce Infection Deaths has this to say about hospital infections:

> Sometimes connecting the dots reveals a grim picture. Several new reports about hospital infections show that the danger is increasing rapidly, and that the federal Centers for Disease Control and Prevention isn't leveling with the public about it... It is common for government regulators to become soft on the industry they are supposed to regulate. A coziness develops...

---

[108] "MRSA and HAI," *Health Watch USA*, http://www.healthwatchusa.org/mrsa/index. html.

where government administrators spend too
much time listening to hospital executives and
not enough time with grieving families.[109]

In front of the hospital in Kansas City, another construction
sign read: "Future site for cancer research." I wondered what exactly were the miracle cures coming out of all of these billion-dol-
lar cancer research centers? I sometimes ask that question of the
medical school students holding plastic buckets at busy intersec-
tions imploring drivers to donate to cancer research. But they of
course don't know of any. Those students would do better to read
Margaret Edson's play *Wit,* or a letter Nora received from a man
whose wife died *after* being "treated" for cancer:

> Dear Nora,
> We met sometime in the early nineties when you
> held a HERS conference in Philadelphia. I was
> there with my wife because she had been "hys-
> terectomized" by Charles Debrovner (notice I
> didn't call him Doctor) in 1989. The pathology
> report post-op stated he removed all healthy
> organs except for a small rice grain fibroid on
> her uterus. The reputed original purpose of
> the operation was to remove a mucinous cyst-
> adenoma on her right ovary. The actual pur-
> pose was Debrovner needed a woman's body so
> three budding doctors could learn how to do
> the procedure. There is a long and gory and
> detailed and damning story involved with this
> tragedy. I'm writing to you because I received
> a letter from your foundation today which is
> the tenth anniversary of her death from pan-
> creatic cancer. I had just lighted a yahrzeit can-
> dle and turned to go over my mail when I saw
> your foundation's letter. I don't know if there

---

[109] McGaughey, Betsy, "CDC's Deadly Mistakes," *Washington Times,* April 15, 2008.

are any studies linking hysterectomies with later deaths due to cancer, but as a physician myself I certainly would bet on that one. I believe the procedure has a definite disastrous effect on the immune system. As a final note, Debrovner knew that I was outside the operating room and had specific orders to confer with me should he feel the need to remove any part of her body beyond the ovarian cyst (which was benign). He also had orders that no resident or intern participate in any part of the operation—I have pictures of the operative site showing three styles of the closing suturing.

Thank you for doing your work,

[name omitted for confidentiality]

A free society requires that those who harm others, no matter what their position in life, are held accountable. Bad doctors give good doctors a black eye when they aren't brought to justice, and it's time for good doctors to end their complicit behavior.

Dr. Lopa Mehta teaches Gross Anatomy at a medical school in Mumbai, India. She was the keynote speaker at HERS' 21st Hysterectomy Conference in Philadelphia. Some of her observations join a growing body of evidence contradicting a connection between medicine and longevity. In *un becoming* the character John Tracey paraphrases Lopa Mehta:

JOHN: Anyway this doctor says that when the poor in India go to the clinic and the doctor tells them they have cancer, there's nothing to do but turn around and go back home to live-out the best life they can. But those who have the money get the treatment, the best the west has to offer. And their statistics, which they've been tracking since the 50s, say the life expectancy for those who get the treatment and those who don't is almost the same.

Why is it that some of us trust doctors more than we trust politicians and car salesmen? Many of the drugs that are designed, approved, marketed, and sold by doctors to unsuspecting people are no better than narcotics sold by the pusher on the street or the toxic snake oils sold by traveling salesmen in the days before medicine dominated our culture. In an article titled "Unproven Cancer Treatments: Hope or Hoax?" Lenore Gelb takes a drug called Cancell to task:

> An example of a claim "too good to be true" is found in the promotional literature for Cancell, a currently popular cancer treatment that looks like a dark brown liquid and is made up of ordinary chemicals including nitric acid, sodium sulfite, potassium hydroxide, sulfuric acid, and catechol. The literature for Cancell states that the product is nontoxic and has no side effects. Although the Cancell booklet says no claims are made for the treatment, it also says that the treatment "digests" cancer cells and then, "the cancer no longer exists." No scientific evidence supports the use of Cancell for any disease, and no data have been submitted to FDA on Cancell's safety or effectiveness. FDA has conducted numerous regulatory investigations of Cancell, and has taken its promoters to court to try to stop its distribution.[110]

Even still, if you search the web for Cancell you can read all sorts of glowing reports on the drug, in the same way that if you search for information on hysterectomy you're likely to find websites that tout the so-called "happy hysterectomy" with testimonials

---

[110] Gelb, Lenore "Unproven Cancer Treatments: Hope or Hoax?" *FDA Consumer Magazine*, March 1992.

from women who are somehow "better than ever" after their sex organs are removed.

With all of the construction going on at the Kansas University Medical Center, there was nowhere for us to protest near the hospital. Throngs of medical students and visitors dodged out of the way of earthmovers and forklifts, as cranes crisscrossed the sky overhead. We papered a few hundred cars in the parking garage and nearby surface lots.

Nora went inside the hospital, taking the elevator up to what she called an "academic floor" of the hospital. She then papered a clinical floor, where women and men sat waiting to be seen by freshly-trained doctors who might've just learned how to perform the prescribed treatment just moments before in a classroom upstairs. Modern medicine gives "on the job training" a whole new meaning when you're the subject.

As Nora slipped pamphlets under office doors, a security guard spotted her. "You looking for the parking lot?" he asked. He then kindly escorted her to our rental car, where I was waiting for her.

There was a performance of *un becoming* by Blue Moon Productions at the Late Night Theatre in Kansas City, Missouri, with the expert help of Crossroads Theatre, playwright Bill Nelson, and director Robert Paisley. It was a superb performance in a wonderful venue. During the talkback, a man in the first row recounted how his wife died on the operating table during a hysterectomy.

Later, Robert and his family hosted a cast party. Several actors and their friends pulled me aside to tell me how hysterectomy had impacted their lives. Actors often don't feel comfortable talking about these issues until the talkbacks are over. Any one of their stories would serve as an appropriate Surgeon General's warning for America's hospitals.

It was from a woman in Kansas that Nora received a letter with this stark report: "There isn't a woman in my church who still has a uterus, and every woman in town attends my church." It was a nearly identical statement to what a woman in Mississippi told Nora. I told this to someone at the party, and she said, "And for every woman you hear about, how many others are there? We probably don't have any idea how big of a problem this is."

THIRTY-SEVEN

The car accident hysterectomy.

Salt Lake City, Utah—Nora W. Coffey

Many women we've spoken with question their faith when a "religious" doctor leads them to an unnecessary operation. Others view what was done to them as the work of darker forces, or even a punishment from God. A woman named Edith in Austria said in an email to HERS, "God doesn't give me any answer. He lets me alone with all these questions." Still others place themselves within the context of a sort of savior complex, viewing their post-operative problems as their "cross to bear." As Stacy in Utah said, "It's a burden I can handle."

Stacy (name changed for confidentiality) was hysterectomized by a doctor who was a fellow Mormon. Stacy knows now the doctor obscured the facts of the operation, and she stood with me in front of the Intermountain Healthcare LDS Hospital, a hospital affiliated with the Church of Jesus Christ of Latter-day Saints.

By that point we were gradually forming a plan to stop unconsented hysterectomy at its source. Stacy's brother-in-law Jim was an attorney, so she arranged for us to talk. I wanted to speak with anyone who could tell us how we might change the law.

"Before the surgery Stacy and I had a lot of fun," Jim said. "I admire her as a wonderful wife and mother...smart, caring. But the moment she got out of surgery I knew she was changed. I recognized it immediately. She just wasn't the person I always knew."

It's a rare gift for a woman to have someone like Jim who understands what hysterectomy did to them. Most hysterectomized women who are struggling to come to grips with the effects of the surgery have no need for someone who tells them they're just as fun, beautiful, or sexy as they were before the surgery. They know they're not. Most women want someone to validate their experiences, not deny their reality. Each day they discover the many ways they're diminished and damaged. It's maddening to know you've been changed but no one else understands, accepts, or validates your reality.

Stacy arrived late, so I began the protest alone. A doctor came out of the hospital to tell me I wouldn't be "allowed." When I didn't leave, he returned inside and called a higher-up. When I also refused the hospital administrator's demands, he stormed away, too.

It was a bitter cold day with strong winds. During one of my warming-up breaks a security guard rushed out of the hospital and aggressively demanded that I go away. "You're not allowed to come back out and protest," he said, "so you better just stay in your car and go home."

"We have a permit to be here," I said.

"I don't really care!" he said. "The hospital doesn't want you here, and you can't to stand out here again."

"But I will," I said, "just as soon as I get warm. As a security guard you should know a person's rights before you threaten to violate them. I suggest that you talk with someone who's familiar with the First Amendment to the Constitution and stop harassing me before I call the police myself."

Certain that he was right, the security guard returned to the hospital in a huff. In a few minutes he was back again, this time with another guy who asked to see the permit. He said he'd like to bring the permit inside to show the hospital administrators.

"Your behavior doesn't exactly give me confidence that I'll ever see the permit again," I said, "so I'll come in with you."

The idea of inviting me inside the hospital was of course completely unacceptable to them. He thought about this for a moment before saying, "I absolutely, positively guarantee we'll be back in 20 minutes. I just want to make a copy of it."

"What are your names?" I asked. I wrote them down, saying, "Okay, I'll let you have it for 20 minutes."

As they walked away, I resumed protesting. When I got cold again I went back to the car. As I warmed up, the same two men returned. Not only did they bring the permit as promised, they brought hot cocoa, crackers, and a few sticks of gum. It was a strange peace offering, but it did make me smile. Only a short while before they were yelling at me. Now here they stood with big, jovial smiles telling me I was welcome, and would I please accept their apologies on behalf of LDS Hospital? We talked for a while, I gave them pamphlets, and they returned inside, reading them as they walked away.

By that time, Stacy showed up. In spite of the frigid temperatures, there was good foot traffic coming from the hospital parking lot. We got information into the hands of pretty much everyone who came and went. Very few people said anything to us, but no one refused the information.

Stacy had never participated in a protest before. She was tentative at first but seemed to grow taller and emboldened as the day wore on. After a while I saw her walking right up to doctors. "I'd like you to read this," she'd say, handing them a pamphlet. I watched her keep an eye on one of the female doctors all the way to the front door, the doctor reading the pamphlet as she entered the hospital.

The next morning I checked my email while the hotel maintenance crew shoveled snow into the swimming pool beneath the window of my room. One of the emails was from a woman who lived in Utah. What follows are the first three messages of our email exchange:

> Her: i HAVE BEEN REFUSED HEALTH IN-
> SURANCE BECAUSE A ULTRASOUND RE-
> QUIRED PRIOR TO A KIDNEY TRANSPLANT
> DONATION REVEALED A FIBROID TUMOR
> IN MY UTERUS. NOW TO BE ACCEPTED FOR
> INSURANCE, THE INSURANCE COMPANY
> WANTS ME TO HAVE A HYSTERECTOMY!!
> i HAVEN'T HAD ANY ADVERSE SYMPTOMS
> OR AWARENESS OF THE TUMOR. DO YOU
> HAVE ANY SUGGESTIONS OR INFORMA-
> TION –OR RECOMMENDATIONS OF GYNO-
> COLOGIST IN THE AREA?
>
> Me: I would like to help you. I think this is an
> outrageous reason to deny you medical insur-
> ance. Are you the kidney donor or recipient?
> Has the transplant taken place, and if so when?
> You asked for recommendations of doctors in
> your area. Where do you live?
>
> Her: My husband needed a kidney in May of
> 2005, I went through all the testing to donate.
> He died before we could do the transplant. It
> is rigorous testing. I passed all with flying col-
> ors. But the last ultrasound, which I never even
> saw or discussed showed a fibroid tumor. I did
> not even know about it until the insurance
> found the record and denied me. I have never
> had any adverse symptoms, and I am in meno-
> pause. However, the insurance informed me
> that I would need to have a hysterectomy and
> be cleared by the doctors before they would ac-
> cept me. I do not want to have a hysterectomy
> just for insurance. I have found a web site that
> discusses other treatments for fibroids. Because
> of my husband's death, I can purchase Cobra
> insurance until June 2006. I was just trying to
> purchase insurance because I am only 49 and
> cannot get Medicare.

Just when I think I've heard it all, there's another unbelievable story. I'd heard about "car accident hysterectomies," to treat benign fibroids found during a routine MRI on a woman taken to the hospital after a car accident. I'd heard about "allergy hysterectomies," to treat minor stress incontinence during seasonal, allergy-related coughing fits. But I'd never heard of a "kidney transplant hysterectomy," to treat an asymptomatic fibroid spotted during a routine radiology study prior to a kidney transplant, even though the woman's husband died before the transplant could occur. Clearly, doctors will stop at nothing to do this to women. They'll never give it up voluntarily. We'll have to take it away from them.

An asymptomatic, benign fibroid means that it's not causing any problems and it poses no medical risk. It obviously requires no treatment, let alone removing her female organs. And because this woman was menopausal, she already had all the fibroids she was ever going to have. But the medical industry increasingly characterizes menopause as a disease.

Just as menarche is the beginning of menstruation and signals the first possibility of fertility, menopause is the end of menstruation and fertility. It's no more of a disease than menarche. If good health is the goal, it's important for women to be educated about these issues. The goal should be to avoid treatment with education. The information about menopause presented below should be published on every hospital website and provided to women by doctors.

Women who are curious about how soon they'll be menopausal can request a simple, routine test to measure the amount of follicle stimulating hormone (FSH) in a blood sample. A written order from a doctor is needed for an FSH test, which can then be taken to any hospital hematology lab to have the blood drawn. The result will then be sent to the physician who gave you the order, who will then provide you with the results of the test.

It's important that the blood is drawn the first or second day after menstruation begins. If it's drawn at any other time, the results are unreliable. Although the test can't determine the exact date menopause will begin, many women—especially if they're experiencing heavy bleeding, irritability, or hot flashes—find it helpful to know whether these symptoms will soon end or if menopause is still a few years off. It's particularly helpful information for someone considering a surgery like myomectomy, to remove fibroids.

Women develop all the fibroids they're going to have by the age of 40. They often have a rapid growth spurt just before menopause, and tend to slowly and gradually shrink to a negligible size and calcify after menopause. By telling women roughly when menopause will begin, the FSH test can keep them out of the operating room by telling them if when their fibroids will no longer be an issue. Here's a chart that explains how to interpret the results of the FSH test:

If:	Then:
FSH is over 40	you're post-menopausal
FSH is 30-40	menopause will begin very soon
FSH is 20-30	menopause will begin in a few years
FSH is under 20	menopause will begin in more than a few years

Perimenopause is the time prior to the end of menstruation when the ovaries produce less estrogen (known as female hormones, though they're present in both women and men), increase the production of androgens (known as male hormones, but, again, are present in both men and women), and stop producing follicles. When the ovaries stop producing follicles, conception is no longer possible.

Although the ovaries of postmenopausal women no longer produce follicles and women develop all of the fibroids they'll ever have long before menopause, postmenopausal ovarian cysts are common. They are, however, generally benign, and are a natural function of the ovaries. It's important to keep in mind that if the cyst is benign it's nothing to be alarmed about. The difference between a benign and malignant cyst can be easily demonstrated with an ultrasound.

Ovarian cysts with all the features of ovarian cancer warrant removal of the cyst to determine if it's benign or malignant. If an ovarian cyst is solid with papillary projections and there's a significant amount of free fluid in the pelvis, it has a high probability of being malignant. Ovarian cysts that do not display all of these features have a very high probability of being benign. When in doubt, a color-flow Doppler test (similar to an ultrasound) of the blood supply to both ovaries will measure the resistive index. When the resistive index is normal in both ovaries, you can be sure that whatever kind of cyst it is, it's highly likely that it's benign.

Many women are told that after hysterectomy they'll be thrust into an immediate surgical menopause. This is a myth. A menopausal woman has a functioning uterus and ovaries. A woman whose female organs have been removed doesn't have the benefit of the natural hormones and other substances the uterus and ovaries produce. Although the uterus isn't known to produce hormones, it produces hormone-like substances, such as prostaglandin and prostacyclin, which is responsible for a reduced risk of coronary disease in women.

With the medicalization of menopause, menopause centers have sprung up in hospitals and clinics all over the country. They're often funded by and affiliated with drug manufacturers or compounding pharmacies that produce what they refer to as hormone replacement therapy (HRT).

HRT is an oxymoron, because nothing can replace the functions of the ovaries. If a woman with her sex organs intact doesn't take hormones after menopause, she'll continue to produce all the hormones she needs. If she takes hormones, the drugs will suppress the ovaries' ability to produce hormones and the ovaries will atrophy. Whether by surgical removal, chemical destruction, or atrophy, the correct medical term for the loss of ovarian function at any age is castration.

THIRTY-EIGHT

Acupuncture, diet, exercise, reiki...for endocrine balance.

Tulsa, Oklahoma—Nora W. Coffey

Over the years I've noticed that people from different parts of the country talk differently about hysterectomy. Women from the middle part of the country are often exceedingly polite, deferential, and more cautious when they call HERS. If there isn't an appointment available for a couple of weeks, they often say, "That's okay, thank you," and hang up. Even if they're scheduled for surgery the next day, it's not polite for them to insist on speaking with someone the way that some women from New York or Los Angeles might. Many of the women who hang up without saying goodbye are the ones who are struggling the most.

A woman from Oklahoma City I spoke with called HERS because she was desperate for relief from depression, joint pain, hot flashes, weight gain, and insomnia following hysterectomy. "I don't want to take hormones," she said. "Isn't there anything else I can do?"

Bone, joint, and muscle pain are common after hysterectomy and can range from mild to debilitating. The back, buttock, hips, thumbs, and wrists are the most common areas for severe pain. Particularly in women who are very thin, the pain can become debilitating around the ischial tuberosity bones (prominent bones in the buttocks). This stems from the loss of fat pads after hysterectomy, which can make it difficult or impossible to sit. The standard medical recommendation for this kind of pain is cortisone injections into the joints or back. While cortisone may provide temporary relief, it's a dangerous steroid that causes softening of the bones, especially when used repeatedly. Also, "cortisone flares" are common, which occur when the drug crystallizes and causes pain that is often worse than the pain it is often intended to alleviate.

Ice can provide significant pain relief by reducing inflammation and numbing the nerve pathways. It should be applied in an icepack (not directly against the skin) wrapped in a thin towel. Ice can provide pain relief for as long as 24 hours. It shouldn't be applied for more than 20 minutes at a time, but can be frequently reapplied.

"There's no cure for the pain," I said to the caller from Oklahoma City, "but ice helps, and acupuncture is often helpful."

"Did you just say acupuncture?" she asked. She gradually warmed up to the idea after we talked about it, though, and some time later she called to say she found an acupuncturist in Oklahoma who helped her get temporary relief.

Acupuncture treatments can help relieve premenstrual syndrome (PMS), depression, insomnia, joint and muscle pain, muscle cramps, dry eyes, migraines, irregular or heavy menstrual bleeding, pelvic pain, hormonal imbalance, and polycystic ovarian syndrome (PCOS).

PCOS, also called Stein-Leventhal Syndrome, occurs when the ovaries produce a large number of cysts (generally more than 15 cysts in any one ovary). Although they're benign and physiologic (functional), they don't completely resolve after menstruation.

Because these cysts are filled with hormones, particularly androgens, women with PCOS have unusual facial and body hair growth, as well as thinning scalp hair in a male pattern.

A hallmark of PCOS is a heavy vertical line of hair from the navel to the pubis. The high level of hormones can also play havoc with mood and cause heavy menstruation. It rarely causes significant medical problems though, and most women find the biggest challenge to be their change of appearance.

PCOS is confirmed with an ultrasound and is present in about 5-10% of women of childbearing age and about 25% of premenopausal women. It appears to be hereditary. It's most common in inactive, overweight women. Although acupuncture won't completely stop the development of multiple cysts, it can help mediate the symptoms. Hormone agonists (drugs that block the production of hormones) are the most common treatment, but they can also play havoc with the endocrine system.

Acupuncturists can't correct these problems after hysterectomy and castration, because the ovaries and uterus have been removed. As the caller from Oklahoma City learned, although even temporary relief was welcome, in the best case scenario a few weeks of relief is the most a hysterectomized woman can hope for. The treatments must be repeated to have any benefit.

Many HMOs and insurance companies will pay for acupuncture if the treatment is provided by a doctor. Of the three schools of acupuncture—Chinese, Japanese, and the English school—Japanese acupuncture seems to work best for hysterectomized women and for endocrine imbalance in women who haven't had the surgery. I recommend that women find an acupuncturist who uses disposable needles, or they can buy their own. Mark D. Seem is an acupuncturist in New York City who is particularly good at treating endocrine imbalance and post-hysterectomy problems.

Acupressure may also be effective in relieving symptoms. Acupressure uses the same points on the body as acupuncture, but instead of needles the gentle pressure of hands and feet is used to release muscular tension and promote circulation. Although not quite as effective as acupuncture, it can relieve some of the same symptoms and you can learn how to apply acupressure to yourself.

Similar to acupuncture and acupressure, reiki promotes healing through deep relaxation and the opening of energy blockages. Reiki is distinctly different from acupuncture and acupressure because a reiki practitioner places his or her hands on or just above a particular part of the person's body to improve the flow of energy and relieve pain. HERS has counseled a small number of women who use reiki who have found it to be beneficial.

Exercise and diet play an important role for hysterectomized women. The average weight gain is 25 pounds in the first year after the surgery. Any weight bearing or aerobic exercise is beneficial, particularly jumping rope. It strengthens the muscles and is an excellent cardiovascular workout.

Another common problem post-hysterectomy is adhesions that cause pulling or pain in the pelvis. Adhesions often develop after pelvic surgery, whether the surgery is exploratory laparoscopy, laparotomy, or a C-section. They also develop from pelvic infections, IUDs, D&Cs, and the scraping of endometrial implants in the pelvis. An effective way to break up adhesions and relieve pelvic pain is with yoga exercises (see the exercises by Sheila Iyengar in the back of B. K. S. Iyengar's *Light On Yoga*[111]) or gentle massage. If a pelvic infection or inflammation is present, deep massage

[111] Iyengar, B. K. S., *Light On Yoga*, Knopf, 1995.

should be avoided, because it may increase pain, cause irritation, and worsen the inflammation.

In Tulsa, I stayed in a historic hotel with a comfortable lounge. One night during my stay, the bartender leaned across the bar toward me and asked what I was doing in town. When I told him, the smile on his face vanished and he leaned back against the carved walnut and marble counter behind him, polishing a glass. After a while, without looking up, he said, "My mother had a hysterectomy."

"What do you remember?" I asked.

"Well, she was never the same after that!" he said more loudly than he wanted to, remembering he had other customers. He leaned close again, saying more quietly, "She never really recovered from it." And that was the last we spoke of it.

When I ask women I'm counseling from "the OK state" how they're doing, they usually say, "I'm fine," even if they're not sure how they'll make it through another day. Except for the doctor who hysterectomized them, most of the women I counsel in this part of the country haven't talked about hysterectomy with anyone but me. When gynecologists respond to their long list of problems after the surgery by telling them all the other women in their practice are happy, they tend not to argue.

THIRTY-NINE

"See not, hear not, know not."

Richmond, Virginia—Nora W. Coffey

Our Richmond protest was held at the Medical College of Virginia Commonwealth University (VCU). Dorothy was in front of the hospital, Susan and Eunita were across the street, and I was in front of the medical school where there was a lot of foot traffic.

In general the medical students were annoyed to see us out there. Some of them took our materials, but most of them did their best to avoid us. They seemed uncomfortable with being educated outside of their classrooms.

Medical students are taught that their power depends on keeping medical information within the confines of the medical establishment. The more specialized they become, the wider the divide between what they know and we know. The greater that divide, the more power accrues to them. When we learn what they know, they wield less power over us. So our pamphlets were a direct threat to their monopoly on information.

The HERS mandate is:
> to provide information about the alternatives to and consequences of hysterectomy that are requisite to informed consent. The HERS Foundation is an independent non-profit international women's health education organization. It provides full, accurate information about hysterectomy, its adverse effects and alternative treatments.

The VCU Obstetrics and Gynecology website also talks about education as a fundamental precept of its mission:

> Education is what we are about: education is what makes us different, education is why we are here. Everything we do must be measured by its contribution to education. Service to the community is an integral component of our education mission. High quality, innovative healthcare for the women of Virginia is fundamental to our effort to educate the physicians and specialists of the future. Furthermore, research that continuously expands the limits of our knowledge about diseases of women is also a critical component of our education effort. Without cutting edge research, the quality of our education is suspect. Therefore, although service and research are critical in support of education, it is education that is our top priority. Service and research must be measured by their contribution to this primary mission of education.[112]

They say eleven times in eight sentences that their mission is "education."

Many of the students passing by our protest went to extraordinary lengths to avoid us. Some jumped over a large wall to get around us, sometimes even running to avoid us. "First Do No Harm," that infamous, hollow oath gynecological students repeat when they receive their white coats, might as well be replaced with "See Not, Hear Not, Know Not."

Of the thousands of students who passed by that week, only a handful stopped to take information. One young woman paused long enough to say, as though apologizing for her fellow students, "Thank you. Really. Thank you."

---

[112] http://www.obgyn.vcu.edu/department/mission.htm.

At one point I thought, 'Nothing unusual so far. All we need now is an angry security guard. And, here he comes now.'

The security yelled at Dorothy and Susan so menacingly they moved to the opposite corner, although they had every right to stand where they were. When he approached me, barking that it was time for us to leave, I told him we'd do no such thing.

He bared his teeth and growled, "You have to leave here now! You're on private property!" He actually bumped into me with his belly and stooped over so we were nose-to-nose. I could feel his breath on my face.

I took a step back, saying, "You have no right to treat people this way. We're on public property."

"This sidewalk," he snarled, taking a step toward me again, "belongs to the hospital, and all those buildings belong to the university, and all those other sidewalks. You're not allowed to be on any of it."

"I understand that's what you believe," I replied, "but you're mistaken. This is a public sidewalk, and our protest is completely legal."

As far as the university was concerned, the Supreme Court has ruled in favor of free speech on university campuses, saying that speech activities are vital to university life. And because the university is state-affiliated, our rights were even more clear.[113] We were always careful to either obtain a permit or get something in writing where permits weren't required. Still the security guard ranted and raved before storming back inside.

Richmond was cold, but the weather didn't slow Eunita down. When one person refused to take a pamphlet from her, it

[113] Gora, Goldberger, Stern, and Halperin, *The Right To Protest: The Basic ACLU Guide to Free Expression*, Southern Illinois University Press, 1991.

only made her more determined to put one into the hands of the next person she saw.

Many women hiked long distances in that frigid weather or drove far out of their way to get information from us. "Every woman in my family has had a hysterectomy except me," one woman told me. We talked for a while, then she asked for extra pamphlets to bring home. "I'll be the first one in my family not to get one," she said.

On the fourth day of the protest, Dorothy set two protest signs and a stack of pamphlets down and went inside to warm up. She was away for no more than five minutes, but while she was gone the security guard took them. Richmond was only one of two protest sites where this happened. Undeterred, Dorothy got a new sign out of the trunk of the rental car, a new stack of pamphlets, and barely missed a beat.

Many interesting men and women joined the protests around the country. It's a shame we couldn't document all of their experiences in their own voices. The following diary entry tells what the protest was like from Dorothy's perspective:

> A very young woman with a baby and another little child hurried by me, then hesitated and came back for some literature. She wanted to know just what a hysterectomy was. I explained that hysterectomy is the removal of the uterus, and she said, "Oh, no, that's not what I had. I just had my reproductive organs taken out. I'm going back now for my after-operation checkup." Just what organs the doctor removed isn't known. It is unconscionable that a doctor would not take the time to explain to her not only what her choices were but the complications of each choice—even if that meant giv-

ing her a short course in a woman's anatomy. What bothers me more is that when I tell this story to people the response I receive is usually either a slight giggle or disdain over a woman who doesn't know her own body. Yet, I wonder if they really understand their own bodies or what's more important whether they understand that practicing doctors have a responsibility to their patients... I also remember a group of med students brushing by me and loudly indicating that I'm not only intruding but I do not realize the importance of the hysterectomy in "saving the woman's life." The next day the situation changed. Several of these same students came back for literature telling me they must read up on the information for a special conference that was being scheduled. How wonderful to know the impact our message made. Along these same lines a woman surgeon stood reading the list of hysterectomy complications from the literature handout. She remarked that she performed a large number of hysterectomies... What surprised me most was the mentality of two medical school teachers adamantly opposing my presence with loud, vulgar remarks saying that if women can have an abortion then they can have a hysterectomy. And then there was this wonderful, older man who just stood there for the longest time listening and nodding his head in agreement. When he discovered we were all volunteers, he contributed three dollars to our cause.

FORTY

Pelvic inflammatory disease; the fallacy of informed consent.

Los Angeles, California—Rick Schweikert

The art deco main building of the Los Angeles County & University of Southern California Hospital (also known as County USC) was used in the daytime television show *General Hospital.* The melodrama we ran into with County USC's security guard could've landed him a cameo role. The treatment one of our fellow protestors received there a few years earlier, however, was straight out of a horror movie.

Nancy (name changed for confidentiality), a Los Angeles attorney, was experiencing severe abdominal pain. She thought it was her appendix, but a CT scan revealed pelvic inflammatory disease (PID).

PID generally begins as an infection in the fallopian tubes (called a hydrosalpinx) and is most commonly caused by intrauterine contraceptive devices (IUDs), when a woman doesn't change her tampons often enough, or it can be sexually transmitted. Bacteria normally found in the vagina, as well as strep or staph infections, travel from the vagina into the cervix, then into the uterus, and from there into the fallopian tubes. Diagnostic and surgical procedures in the vagina or pelvis can also cause infection.

Although her infections could've been treated non-invasively, the doctor insisted that surgery was necessary to save Nancy's life. Nancy did what she could to protect herself, modifying the consent form and adding a few pages of her own. More specifically, she made it clear she wasn't consenting to hysterectomy.

If the source of her problem indicated that any organs should be removed, she wanted to make that decision when she woke up from the anesthesia. Nonetheless, the doctor removed her uterus and ovaries against her wishes. Nancy was now hysterectomized and castrated because of the doctors' failure to diagnose and promptly treat an infection in her pelvis.

In addition to being a lawyer herself, Nancy's mother was a nurse and her sister was a doctor, and both stood at her side throughout this medical fiasco. "If this can happen to me," Nancy said, "then no woman is safe."

To determine the correct antibiotics to treat an infection, the doctor must first make a culture of the infection. Antibiotics can skew culture results, so it's important to wait until the presence of any antibiotics is gone before a culture is done.

Here's an email HERS received from Nancy regarding the continued problems she experienced after the hysterectomy:

> I wish to thank you for your professional and kind support during my months of physical and emotional recovery… For the past month, I was placed on a 4 mg per day dosage of oral Estrace [an exogenous hormone]. Two days ago, I experienced a TIA [transient ischemic attack— an episode of insufficient blood supply to the brain], which lasted approximately 35 minutes. During this time, I suffered vision impairment coupled with an inability to speak, recognize, or even understand written language. I was seen by my primary physician who immediately reduced the estrogen prescribed by a different physician. Now, I am undergoing MRIs, carotid artery ultrasounds, and will be seen by a neurologist. Suffice to say, once again, I do not know who to trust or what to do. This nightmare just seems to go on indefinitely.

Nancy's story also demonstrates the ineffectiveness of the current hysterectomy consent form process. It protects hospitals and doctors, not patients.

Nora was asked to support legislation for a standardized hysterectomy consent form in the state of New York. She explained that she wasn't able to support it because, like the California hysterectomy consent form, the proposed New York form would be used by hospitals and doctors to keep women from pursuing medical malpractice lawsuits. They did succeed in developing a hysterectomy consent form that is more comprehensive than most, but it isn't mandatory, and more than 38,000 women continue to be needlessly hysterectomized and castrated each year in New York.[114] If you search for the New York model hysterectomy consent form, you're not likely to find it. My online search for it was in vain. In fact, the only consent form I found on the New York State Department of Health's website was for Medicaid recipients that lists sterilization as the only consequence of hysterectomy.

Medicaid consent forms themselves vary from state to state. Most states use a form called something like "Acknowledgement of Hysterectomy Information," and it says, "The reason for performing the hysterectomy and the discomforts, risks and benefits associated with the hysterectomy have been explained to me and all my questions have been answered to my satisfaction prior to the surgery." But the person giving consent has no way of knowing if they've been fully informed. They only know what they've been told.

---

[114] Total New York population 19,306,183, women 51.5% = 9,942,684, 76.6% over 18 years old = 7,616,095. Hysterectomy rate in New York 5/1,000 = 38,080. "US Census Bureau, State & County QuickFacts, 2006." Also see, Kolata, Gina, "Rate of Hysterectomies Puzzles Experts," *New York Times*, September 20, 1988.

Medicaid consent forms also generally contain a provision called "Waiver of Acknowledgment and Surgeon's Certification." This is the place where the surgeon signs the form on behalf of the woman whose signature the surgeon determines is unnecessary because of "a life threatening emergency." While it's sometimes critical for a qualified person to make decisions for us when we're not capable of making them for ourselves, this "emergency" caveat lends itself to abuse. About half of the women who call HERS were hysterectomized during exploratory surgery or surgery to remove a benign cyst or fibroid. Once a woman is unconscious on the operating table with her abdomen opened up, the courts have deemed that any reasonable physician could be expected to perform a hysterectomy without waking her up and asking for consent to remove her sex organs.

The consent forms often state the kind of surgery to be performed, such as "exploratory surgery, possible removal of an ovarian cyst, and possible TAH/BSO." During exploratory surgery, when a surgeon uses a laparoscope (a tube-like instrument inserted through the abdomen to provide a view of the internal organs), only the doctor and anyone looking at the monitor attached to the camera on the laparoscope can see the image of what's inside the pelvis. Afterwards, there's no one else to confirm or refute what the surgeon says he or she saw. Only after the tissue or organs are removed and sent to the pathology lab, where a microscopic exam is conducted by a pathologist, can it be determined whether or not you have the condition the surgeon says you had. You can obtain a copy of the pathology report from a hospital's medical records department, but by then it's too late. Women fax their pathology reports to HERS, and we help them understand the medical terms, but it's usually not until then they discover for the first time the hysterectomy was unwarranted.

When the surgeon writes onto the consent form "possible TAH/BSO"—total abdominal hysterectomy and bilateral salpingo oophorectomy (castration)—the word "possible" is a caveat that gives the surgeon the legal consent he or she needs to remove your uterus and ovaries. Throughout 25 years of reading the medical records of women who call HERS, Nora has yet to see a hysterectomy consent form that effectively indemnifies or informs women prior to surgery. Wilton H. Bunch put it this way:

> In teaching hospitals, the task [of getting the consent form signed] is assigned to the most junior resident who has little or no knowledge of the procedure or the complications. The law is fulfilled, but the intention is thwarted... In a study of 100 patients questioned 2 to 5 days after surgery, it was reported that 27% of the patients did not even know what organ had been operated on... There have been no winners in this war.[115]

Bunch details the sketchy history of informed consent rising from the murky depths of what he calls the "professional standard." The professional standard rule, Bunch tells us, says doctors should "tell the patient and the family the amount of information that other competent surgeons would have disclosed." In other words, let history be our guide to the future. It's not about providing the information women need to make informed decisions, it's about only providing as much information as other doctors might provide. Bunch says the result is a situation where "human experimentation became mainstream...to test hypotheses."

---

[115] Bunch, Wilton H., "Informed Consent," *Clinical Orthopaedics and Related Research*, September 2000.

I was told that California passed Senate Bill 835, requiring a more comprehensive hysterectomy consent form. It was said to be the prototype hysterectomy consent form that inspired similar legislation in New York. But like New York's consent form, I couldn't find it online. So I contacted the Medical Board of California. Their response was, "We are unable to locate the bill you specified." What they provided was the California Health and Safety Code 1690-1691, which requires doctors to obtain verbal and written informed consent.[116] It's a code—a regulation—but it's not a law. It's unenforceable and easily disregarded.

No state, including California, has a law on the books that puts the burden of proof on the surgeon to warrant that they provided full disclosure of the well-documented adverse effects of removing the uterus or ovaries. The only hysterectomy consent I could find that is required by California law is for Medicaid and MediCal recipients. The disclosure is limited to sterilization, and it's deemed unnecessary when "the hysterectomy was performed under a life-threatening emergency in which [the surgeon] determined prior acknowledgment was not possible."[117]

Clearly, the current accepted "standard of care" is defined by the doctors who perform hysterectomies. They establish a norm for the functions of the female organs. Any variation from that norm is then considered abnormal, and treatment is prescribed.

---

[116] Webmaster@mbc.ca.gov, email to Rick Schweikert "Re: Senate Bill 835," December 12, 2006. California Safety Code 1691 says: "The failure of a physician and surgeon to inform a patient by means of written consent, in layman's language and in a language understood by the patient of alternative efficacious methods of treatment which may be medically viable, when a hysterectomy is to be performed, constitutes unprofessional conduct within the meaning of Chapter 5 (commencing with Section 2000) of Division 2 of the Business and Professions Code."
[117] U.S. Department of Health and Human Services, Centers for Medicare and Medicaid Services, Title 42 Code of Federal Regulations, § 441.255.

The American College of Obstetricians and Gynecologists (ACOG) creates "criteria sets" for anything that falls outside the norm. These include menorraghia, or heavier than normal menstrual bleeding. A woman with heavier monthly flow than others might be told she has a disease, and treatment of minor variations becomes the accepted standard of care. It's the fox guarding the hen house. It means that any anatomical deviation from a hypothetical average, including benign variations that require no treatment at all, might be used as justification for a damaging, life-altering surgery.

Many doctors and researchers have written about this troubling situation. Arthur Caplan, chair of the department of Medical Ethics at the University of Pennsylvania, told Judy Foreman of the *Los Angeles Times* that the informed consent process "has become more of a shield than a doorway."[118] And one week later, Foreman reported the following:

> More than 90% of hysterectomies in the U.S. are not done because of cancer, but because a woman has fibroids, endometriosis, abnormal bleeding, or a prolapsed or fallen uterus—all conditions for which less drastic surgery or non-surgical treatments are available.
> "Women are not told enough about the downsides of hysterectomy and the alternatives so they can make a truly informed decision," said Dr. Mitchell Levine, a Cambridge, Mass., gynecologist.[119]

---

[118] Foreman, Judy, "More Than Just A Patient's Signature," *Los Angeles Times*, August, 8 2005.
[119] Foreman, Judy, "When Does Hysterectomy Go Too Far?" *Los Angeles Times*, August 15, 2005.

Clearly, California women aren't sufficiently informed about the effects of hysterectomy, and the California Department of Health Services appears to be oblivious to what's at stake. The California Patients' Guide (www.calpatientguide.org) discusses your right to sue the doctor for "failure to get your informed consent":

> If your physician fails to get proper informed consent, this is considered negligence and may be the basis for a malpractice lawsuit. If you think that this has happened to you, immediately consult an attorney who specializes in medical malpractice. The statute of limitations (the time within which the law allows lawsuits to be filed) for medical malpractice is one year from the time you knew or should have known that malpractice had been committed.[120]

But as Nancy found out, medical malpractice lawsuits are very difficult to bring and even more difficult to win. Nancy was unable to bring a lawsuit. Experts agreed she was harmed, but they refused to testify for her because state law provides an exception: the "reasonable physician standard." Any reasonable physician might've done the same thing in a similar situation, so even if Nancy was unreasonably harmed, the doctor who harmed her isn't necessarily culpable. Can you imagine any other profession where a crime is overlooked because the criminal's colleagues commit similar crimes? The following is from Lawyers.com, (emphasis added):

---

[120] *The California Patient's Guide Your Health Care Rights and Remedies*, "IV. Your Right to Informed Consent," Consumer Watchdog. *Cobbs v. Grant*, 8 Cal. 3d 229, 502 P.2d 1, 104 Cal. Rptr. 505 (1972) established that a person may bring an action for battery in the absence of informed consent, and *Thor v. Superior Court*, 5 Cal. 4th 725, 855 P.2d 375, 21 Cal. Rptr. 2d 357 (1993) reaffirmed the basic and "fundamental right" even when a refusal of the proposed medical treatment may cause or hasten death.

> Generally, to win a medical malpractice case, you must have expert medical testimony that **no** reasonable health care provider would have done what yours did… While state law generally determines how negligence is defined, the "standard of care" is generally **defined by the medical community**. It's not the measure of what is optimum care or even the measure of what an expert thinks should have been done in hindsight. The issue is whether any reasonable physician **could have done** what the doctor in question did.[121]

Many people ask us why politicians pass such toothless laws regarding something as critical as informed consent for major surgery. There isn't a short answer, but the campaigns of politicians are often funded by medical industry profits, and reliable information is as difficult for politicians to find as it is for women who are trying to make decisions about their health.

If you're a politician interested in working on hysterectomy consent form legislation, you might ask your aides to search for some "standard" of what women need to be told prior to surgery. In their search, your aides might land on the website of the American College of Surgeons. It sounds legitimate enough, so your aides wander around the ACS website and find their online pamphlet titled "About Hysterectomy." When they do, they can temporarily avoid stepping onto a landmine of bad information by sticking with, "Severe complications and even death occasionally occur with this operation." That's certainly something women need to know. In that same paragraph, ACS even provides an accurate description of the location of the uterus: "The uterus is located

---

[121] "Medical Malpractice FAQs," *Lawyers.com*, http://medical-malpractice.lawyers. com/Medical-Malpractice-FAQs.html.

between the ureters (small tubes which transport urine from the kidneys to the bladder) on each side, the urinary bladder in front, and the rectum behind." At least now your aides can ask the question, "If the uterus sits between these and is removed, how does the surgery impact bladder and bowel function when the support of the uterus and its ligaments are severed and the uterus, which supported and separated these organs, is removed?" To which the authors of the ACS website have formulated a response: "All of these structures are subject to injury… It is not sensible," they say, "to have a hysterectomy in order to prevent cancer of the cervix or uterus." That's right, it's insensible for surgeons to do so. But then your aides read on. The writers of the ACS website later tell them, "Hysterectomy usually has no physical effect on your ability to experience sexual pleasure or orgasm… Most women experience an improvement of mood and increased sense of well-being following hysterectomy. For many, relief from fear of pregnancy results in heightened sexual enjoyment following the procedure."[122] I'd like to hear an ACS representative ask the hysterectomized women we protested with in L.A. about the possibility of improved mood and heightened sexual enjoyment after their sex organs were removed. Imagine a website that said, "For many men, relief from fear of getting a woman pregnant results in heightened sexual enjoyment following removal of the penis."

No woman can be said to have consented to hysterectomy unless *the doctor can prove* that she was fully informed of the well-documented alternatives and adverse effects of the surgery. The onus of proof must fall where it belongs—on the doctors who per-

---

[122] "When You Need an Operation…About hysterectomy," *American College of Surgeons*, http://www.facs.org/public_info/operation/hysterectomy.pdf.

form hysterectomies, not on the women whose bodies and lives they destroy.

The hysterectomy recommendation forwarded to me by the Medical Board of California doesn't come anywhere near to providing the information required for consent. It's nothing but a place for an unsuspecting woman to sign her name to protect doctors, hospitals, and clinics. They often don't even give women the consent form until they're in the pre-op waiting area. In some cases, women aren't provided with the consent form until after they're sedated and already on the operating table. Many women have told us their eyeglasses had already been removed by a nurse, and they couldn't make out the words on the consent form they were being asked to sign.

And even if women were given a ten-page consent form listing all of the adverse effects, doctors can say, "You need to sign this, and don't worry about what it says about the consequences. None of that happens to my patients. In no time you'll be a new woman."

We know there's almost always plenty of time to educate women and consider the options, because the surgery is almost never performed for life-threatening conditions. It's very rarely performed in a true emergency situation.

We can't rely on gynecologists to inform women, because they benefit from hysterectomy. Here's a recent email we received that demonstrates how badly women need this information:

> When you get a hysterectomy do you have any menstal cycle at all? If you do what is going on and is there anything rong with the opperstion? Is there any other facts or movies that the public can watch so that we the people can see what

the really is going to go on in the room when the opperstion is perceeding. Thank you for your time!

Her email indicates that she may have had bleeding after the hysterectomy and that she wasn't informed enough to know that menstrual cycles aren't possible without a uterus, but she's reluctant to speak with the doctor and is searching far and wide for answers she can't get anywhere else. She did find HERS though, so she'll at least find the answers to her questions.

And here's part of an email from a woman who made the realization that medicine is the wrong place for trust. She'll have to depend on her own resources to learn what she needs to know.

> Thank you for making that video! I've sent it to my sisters and closest friends. My gyn three years ago told me he would remove a cyst that wouldn't leave on its own, so the day before the surgery, I had to go to the hospital to sign papers and the last paper I signed was the consent form. Thank GOD I read it because I saw, "oophorectomy" and the other word for removing a fallopian tube. I burst into tears and said this is not what I thought was going to happen, there must be a mistake. The nurse whispered to me that this is not the first time this has happened with this doctor and called his office to see if it was a mistake. He gets on the phone himself and tells me it might be a dermoid cyst and he would risk breaking it and causing an infection by merely cutting it out, but that we could reschedule the surgery after we discuss it in his office. Thank GOD again that I had so many people tell me to get a second opinion. The new doctor ordered an x-ray and by the time it was delivered to her office the cyst was gone! She read my records from the first doc-

tor and was baffled. She said that this cyst was too small to even be considered a dermoid cyst and was mystified why he would even consider surgery…

In her article "'Come Again?' Good Medicine Requires Clarity," Deborah Franklin says, "Unfortunately, according to researchers who have been tracking the ways the [informed consent] process unravels, that sort of helpful discussion is too often replaced with a clipboard of legalese and a pen."[123]

A consequence of the misinformation on medical industry websites is women aren't getting the accurate information they need. An example of this is the interactive hysterectomy video tutorial from the Patient Education Institute, Inc. (PEI) of Coralville, Iowa. It's the only hysterectomy "tutorial" recommended on the National Institutes of Health government website (via MedlinePlus).[124] The information it provides is dangerously wrong and unsupported by anatomical fact. The tutorial is marketed to "manage malpractice risk" and "document patient education and informed consent," but the only way women are able to complete the tutorial from start to finish is to answer some of PEI's questions falsely. In other words, only by agreeing with erroneous information are women allowed to complete the hysterectomy lesson and provide consent to hysterectomy. For further reading, visit the HERS Foundation blog "Hysterectomy—The Experts Speak Out,"

---

[123]   Franklin, Deborah, "'Come Again?' Good Medicine Requires Clarity," *New York Times*, January 24, 2006.
[124]   "Hysterectomy," *MedlinePlus*, U.S. National Library of Medicine and the National Institutes of Health, http://www.nlm.nih.gov/medlineplus/hysterectomy.html; "Hysterectomy," *X-Plain.com*, Patient Education Institute, http://www.nlm.nih.gov/medlineplus/tutorials/hysterectomy/htm/index.htm and http://www.patient-education.com/.

featuring the PEI hysterectomy tutorial at hysterectomyinforma-
tion.blogspot.com/.

So what's the solution? Clearly, every woman who's told she
needs a hysterectomy should be provided with accurate information about alternatives and consequences. They need to be able
to listen to the information if they're blind and read it if they're
deaf. The best way to do this is with a video DVD. The video itself,
the printed text of the video, and the printed anatomical drawings
could then be given to each woman to be taken home to discuss
the information with her support network, without the pressure
and distractions of a doctor's office or operating room. It would be
inexpensive and easily implemented. We know, because we did it.

The HERS video "Female Anatomy" provides the minimum information women require to provide informed consent,
and it's available online at hersfoundation.org/anatomy. It's been
viewed by more than half a million people worldwide as of this
writing, and the cost of producing it was nominal...even to a small
non-profit like HERS. The information provided is anatomically
correct, vetted by a professor of Gross Anatomy and Physiology,
gynecologists, and attorneys.

HERS has received countless emails of thanks for the
female anatomy video. Here's a brief sampling:

- I watched the Video. This is the most information I have
  received ever. I believe every Women should be able to
  see this Video before the Medical facility performs a Hysterectomy! It should be mandatory!

- I am scheduled for a subtotal hysterectomy on Jan 8. I
  found this site on Jan 5. THANK GOD! I can't believe I
  almost had a hysterectomy! I am just in SHOCK at what

I am finding out on this site. I thought I had done my research but everything I've read (before this site) encourages this barbaric procedure! I can't believe my doc did not even discuss anything like this to me. And she's a female doc! I am a healthy 35 year-old mom of 2 kids.

- I have shown all my girlfriends the video and am getting them to sign the petition, naturally they are horrified at the changes a hysterectomy can do to a woman and I am living testimony to this.

- I am schedule to have my surgery Aug 15. Thank God I found your information. Thanks for all the information...it was truely a blessing I found it when I did. I am deaf. I am so grateful I could read it and not have to ask someone...perfect for me! Thank you!!!!!!!!!!!!!

- I teach holistic health care classes for women, and I've recently seen the pamphlet and video that your organization creates regarding hysterectomies. It's a great pamphlet and video! How can I get copies of them to give to my clients/students? Keep up the great work educating women/men worldwide !

The need for this information is vast. Every minute of every business day five more women are taken into surgery and their female organs are removed. Here's an anonymous email from a woman in Los Angeles in a situation similar to Nancy's above, which underscores the urgent need for accurate information:

thank you for the website on alternatives to hysterectomis for uterine fibroids. Please also warn your readers about authorization forms for surgery. Some hospitals are forcing and coercing poor and minority women to undergo hysterectomies against their will. Many believe they are

having myomectomies only to find out that the
authorization form was used to give surgeons
an easy out of the procedure.
I am a patient at harbor-ucla ob-gyn clinic,
in torrance california. I was diagnosed with
fibroids at least 5. The largest fibroid is 7 cm
and is located below my uterus. After 3 years, I
have finally been diagnosed with fibroids. three
years later, with no insurance, I have come to
Harbor UCLA...
I am supposed to have surgery August 16 or
19th. However, I am planning on not going
through with the operation. Although I have
educated myself on myomectomy procedures
the only option I am given is hysterectomy. I am
36 years old and desire to have children. I feel
like I am being punished for being without insurance. I was told that if I did not sign an "authorization to perform a hysterectomy" that no
myomectomy surgery would be performed and
that the hospital would stop treating me. I asked
to read the form. The form is a supplement to
the original form for authorization to perform
a surgery. The supplemental form is for a hysterectomy only not for a myomectomy. I con-
tinually refused to sign the form and pointed
out that the form is a supplement which did not
require me to sign it in order to receive benefits
from the hospital. I don't know if they are going to try to make me sign the form in order to
perform the myomectomy.
I should not be forced to have a hysterectomy
UNLESS I am at death's door during the surgery... I don't want to have a hysterectomy. My
future should not end just because I am temporarily poor and uninsured. Many poor and
minority women are being coerced and tricked
into signing these forms at Harbor UCLA

hospital not knowing that they are not consenting to a myomectomy but a HYSTERECTOMY.
if you have any advice, I greatly appreciate it.
More importantly, tell your readers about this
as soon as possible.

It should be criminal for doctors to perform life-altering surgery on women who aren't given the information they need to make informed decisions. It's inhumane, unconstitutional, and it must be made unacceptable, by making it illegal.

FORTY-ONE

The hysterectomy quota.

Louisville, Kentucky—Nora W. Coffey

The following is from a Lexington *Herald-Leader* article by Anna Tong:

... The plaintiff, 38-year-old Connie Grimes, had filed a lawsuit against Guiler in 2003, saying he performed a medically unnecessary oophorectomy. Although she signed a consent form, Grimes said she did not fully understand the consequences of having her ovaries removed at age 31. Grimes is one of six women who filed a lawsuit against Guiler; the cases are being tried separately. Guiler has previously been in the national spotlight because of other lawsuits filed in 2003 alleging he had etched "UK"—for University of Kentucky, his alma mater—on uteri before he removed them. The courtroom atmosphere was emotional after the verdict...[125]

For logistical reasons, I moved the Kentucky protest from Lexington to Louisville. The hotel I stayed at didn't appear to be expecting travelers. I thought about how on Christmas Day most hospitals are as deserted as that hotel. There are of course just as many emergencies on Christmas as any other day, but it's probably the slowest day of the year for hospitals in the U.S.

I've come to think of holidays as Hysterectomy vacations. If most hysterectomies were medically warranted they'd be performed seven days a week, no weekends or holidays off. But

---

[125] Tong, Anna, "Jury sides with Gynecologist," *Lexington Herald-Leader*, July 2, 2008.

doctors don't want to be in a hospital on holidays, and 98% of hysterectomies are elective, which is another way of saying they aren't needed.

A woman I had counseled many years earlier signed up to meet me at the protest, if she was well enough to leave the house. A registered nurse who was married to a doctor, she was nonetheless castrated without her consent.

I stood at an intersection near the Louisville Baptist Hospital and gave out information for about an hour. Between the cold and the lack of foot traffic, I decided to paper the city instead. I put information under the windshield wipers of cars in church parking lots and went into a bookstore that happened to be open.

Along the way, I saw an advertisement claiming that Norton Hospital was Louisville's healthcare leader. When you travel through as many cities as we were that year, the ubiquitous hospital advertisements claiming "We're #1!" get a little absurd. They all perform unnecessary hysterectomies, and we didn't find one that provided women with the information they need to make informed decisions.

And because Norton is a teaching hospital affiliated with the Louisville University Medical School, the school wouldn't attract medical school students in gynecology if they didn't offer those students lots of hands-on surgical training on live women. There's an unspoken quota system in America's medical schools that seems to view women as test animals for medical students, and huge income generators for the hospitals that help train doctors.

The Accreditation Council for Graduate Medical Education (ACGME) says it's "responsible for the accreditation of post-MD medical training programs within the United States...based on established standards and guidelines."[126] The University of Louisville School of Medicine's website publishes statistics for residents receiving training in Obstetrics and Gynecology. These statistics are gathered by the ACGME and represent "a good average" of what incoming resident physicians can expect to perform in their training.

According to the Resident Statistics on the Louisville School of Medicine website, the "average numbers from a recent graduate" are below. The first column is the number of procedures residents may expect to perform, and the second column is the number of procedures they may expect to assist in:

Abdominal Hysterectomy	123	8
Vaginal Hysterectomy	101	8
Laparoscopic Surgery	128	7
Surgical Sterilization	106	17
Spontaneous Deliveries	293	153
Cesarean Deliveries	252	51

These statistics let a student choosing a residency program know what their opportunity will be to "perform" and "assist" in surgeries. And as the Louisville website says, "These numbers are often used as a basis upon which a graduating resident will obtain hospital privileges."[127]

[126] http://www.acgme.org/acWebsite/home/home.asp.
[127] "Resident Statistics," *Department of Obstetrics, Gynecology, and Women's Health*, University of Louisville, http://louisville.edu/medschool/obgyn/residency/statistics.htm. Note: This web page has been subsequently eliminated, and a new "statistics" page with general institution-wide statistics is now available at http://louisville.edu/medschool/obgyn/education/residency-program/statistics.html.

According to the American Medical Association (AMA), "Economic Credentialing is the use of economic criteria unrelated to quality of care or professional competence in determining a physician's qualifications for initial or continuing hospital medical staff membership or privileges."[128] Louisville's statistics appear to be "unrelated to quality of care or professional competence." They only speak of the numbers of surgeries performed, not the outcomes of the surgeries performed on women by residents. Louisville tells residents how many "numbers" of procedures they'll have an opportunity to perform, to give them the best chance of obtaining privileges at the hospital of their choice.

We don't know the direct charges of the hospitals affiliated with the Louisville School of Medicine, but with about $25,000 of direct hospital and doctor charges for each surgery,[129] hysterectomy is a massive revenue stream for most teaching hospitals. It's good for resident careers and hospital bottom lines, but it's not good for the women who undergo the surgeries.

Gynecologists have told me that quotas are well known and talked about, but they generally remain an unwritten practice. One reason that quotas are rarely published, or even referred to as such, is that the stated goal is supposed to be health, not numbers. When choosing a surgeon, you want one who has performed enough surgeries to demonstrate good outcomes. But the goal should always be to avoid surgery if at all possible, not to help a surgeon meet a quota that keeps the revolving doors of medicine spinning.

---

[128] AMA Policy H-230.975, http://www.ama-assn.org/ama/pub/category/10919.html.
[129] HERS Foundation. Conservative estimate of immediate hospital and doctor-related charges. Does not include additional costs incurred for treatment of chronic adverse effects of the surgery.

Follow the money up the chain of command and you'll see who's in a position of power to do something about this, and why it's in their best interests to do nothing. Money is the serpent entwined around the staff of power, otherwise known as the caduceus—the symbol of Aesculapius (the Greek god of medicine), which is the emblem of the AMA.[130]

I recently shared this information from the Louisville website with a gynecologist. He agreed these "numbers" are common. As a sort of explanation, he went on to say that he doesn't always perform his own surgeries. He's a well-known, experienced surgeon who women come to because of his years of experience and expertise, but he rarely tells his patients when a resident will be performing the surgery in his place. Sometimes he's the primary surgeon and a resident assists, and at other times the resident is the primary surgeon and he supervises and assists them. Some gynecologists, he said, don't assist or supervise, and only make a brief appearance in the operating room if they show up at all.

If you suffer complications at the hands of an inexperienced or unskilled resident, you may never learn who performed the surgery unless you file a medical malpractice lawsuit. It might've been a new resident performing their first surgery on you. Furthermore, embedded in the fine print of the standard consent form is a clause giving the surgeon permission to let anyone in the hospital "treat" you. Some consent forms even specify they're teaching hospitals and that interns and residents may assist in or perform the surgery.

Even still, the doctor I spoke with defended this practice because it's necessary, he said, to train future doctors so they'll learn

[130] http://www.ama-assn.org/ama/pub/category/2133.html.

how to perform surgeries. "And," he said, referring to the hospital where he has privileges, "this *is* a teaching hospital, you know."

Soon the residents he allows to perform his surgeries for him will have their own practices. And if those up-and-coming doctors are affiliated with a teaching hospital, they'll be expected to allow other residents to perform surgeries for them. It's a shell game played with women's bodies and women's lives.

If the statistics on the Louisville website for "a recent graduate" are an accurate portrait of what an average student performs, the "average" Louisville Department of Obstetrics, Gynecology, and Women's Health resident performs over one hysterectomy a week and one female castration every other week, during a 4-year residency. Note that medical students we've spoken with across the country report that gynecologists perform on average 4-6 hysterectomies a week.

There are no definitive sources for the cost of hysterectomy, which varies from hospital to hospital, doctor to doctor, and city to city. But as we've said, according to information provided by women to HERS, the total doctor and hospital charges for each hysterectomy performed in the U.S. averages about $25,000.[131] That means that each resident potentially assists in or performs procedures that generate about $5.6 million in hospital revenue for hysterectomy alone. That number doesn't include the 123 castrations, 135 laparoscopic surgeries, the 303 C-sections, the other "GYN Procedures," or any of the "OB Procedures" they perform or assist in.

---

[131] HERS Foundation. Conservative estimate of immediate hospital and doctor-related charges. Does not include additional costs incurred for treatment of chronic adverse effects of the surgery.

"Spontaneous deliveries," as they're referred to in the Resident Statistics (where there is no surgical intervention), are time-consuming for doctors. Women don't need doctors to have babies, but once a doctor gets involved, time is money. Have you ever heard of a baby that didn't come out? It does happen, but only in very rare instances, such as when the placenta happens to block its own exit by attaching to the cervix (placenta previa), making a C-section lifesaving for both the baby and the mother. And when the placenta doesn't detach from the uterine wall (placenta accreta), sometimes a hysterectomy is the only way of saving the mother's life. But placenta previa can often be managed conservatively and occurs in only 1 in 200 pregnancies. Placenta accreta occurs in only 1 in 2,500 pregnancies. Yet Louisville residents performed or assisted in 5 hysterectomies and 7 C-sections for every 10 spontaneous births.

Medical schools provide students with experience performing surgeries so they can earn hospital privileges. From the hospital's perspective, it's profitable to turn the operating room time around as quickly as possible and, like hotels, keep the beds full. In this way they make each other rich and create jobs, which further enhances their power and influence. But there's someone important missing from this discussion.

The stated purpose of medical schools is to produce skilled doctors. Those at the top of the class will probably have the best skills, and those at the bottom will probably have the worst skills and do the most damage. But whether they're skilled or unskilled at what they do, hysterectomy is rarely lifesaving, and none of the women we've spoken with were provided with the information necessary for informed consent. By the very nature of the surgery, hysterectomy is damaging. The surgeon with the best skill still damages women irrevocably each time he or she removes a uterus.

The heading above these "numbers" isn't "The Number Of Women Treated By Louisville Residents," it's simply "Resident Statistics." This discussion is moot without women, but the authors of this website don't say, "The number of women treated who experience good outcomes are often used as a basis upon which a graduating resident will obtain hospital privileges." The words *woman, women, she, her,* or even *person* or *human being* don't appear in the "resident statistics." Here women are only "numbers" and "statistics," or perhaps most dehumanizing of all—"patients."

In the eyes of the medical-industrial establishment, women are no longer human beings. They're merely patients whose rights and identities are stripped from them along with their clothes... and then their female organs.

In Louisville, a bartender told me she was tending bar because her husband—a rookie cop—was unable to find work after he got out of prison for taking the rap for something in his department. As if telling me about her husband freed her up to talk more openly about herself, she then told me about some medical problems she was having and how "everyone" was telling her she should have a hysterectomy. There was no diagnosis, and what she was experiencing appeared to be more of a nuisance than a medical problem. I gave her my card, telling her to call me if she developed any real problems. She said all the women in her family had been hysterectomized. When I told her what women generally report, she followed each adverse effect I listed with, "My mom has that real bad," or, "Oh yeah, they all have back problems," and, "Yeah, I heard you can't feel anything down there after it," and

"One of them couldn't get out of bed for almost a year, and she still doesn't walk very good."

The blood is on the hands of doctors. But hospitals are finding a way around that too. They're investing in the Da Vinci robot surgery machines. With this device, their hands will be clean as they play the video game known as remote surgery.[132] Medical students doing their OB/GYN rotations have described how surgeons wager who can get the "fastest time" performing a hysterectomy. It's no wonder so many of the women who call HERS come out of operating room with severed ureters, lacerated bladders and bowels, and hideously disfiguring apron-like pelvic incisions.

Intuitive Surgical, which manufacturers Da Vinci robots, recently published its 2008 second quarter earnings report:

> … Our overall gynecologic procedure business registered both the largest sequential percentage growth as well as the largest absolute procedure growth for the quarter. This growth was led by da Vinci Hysterectomy... we continue to expect this procedure to grow at least 150% this year from a base of approximately 13,000 procedures perform last year.[133]

The article refers to robotic hysterectomy as "DVH," in the same way that doctors refer to amputating the uterus and cervix as TAH (total abdominal hysterectomy) and LAVH (laparoscopically-

---

[132] "Robot Surgery: Like Playing a Video Game!" *Cosmetic Surgery Insider*, Tuesday, September 23, 2008: "Gamers, check it out! You have the manual dexterity necessary to become a top surgeon! Using a robot, no less. Says a top surgeon: 'Using the da Vinci surgical robot is almost like paying a video game, like Play Station 3.' So declares Michael Hibner, M.D., director of gynecological surgery at St. Joseph's Hospital and Medical Center in Phoenix."

[133] Intuitive Surgical, Inc., "Q2 2008 Earnings Call Transcript," *Seeking Alpha,* July 22, 2008.

assisted vaginal hysterectomy). Using acronyms and medical double-
speak allows doctors to cloak what they do in scientific language.

As I was composing this chapter, I heard an underwriting
ad for St. Francis Medical System on WHYY, Philadelphia's public
radio station and my local National Public Radio (NPR) affiliate.
The ad was in the voice of an ethereal woman telling the public all
about the Da Vinci surgical robot.

NPR doesn't accept "advertising," per se, though it's sometimes difficult to distinguish an ad on any commercial radio station from corporate underwriting for NPR programming. NPR's
website says it has become "a dominant intellectual force in American life and a primary source of news for millions."[134] WHYY tells
advertisers that listeners "support that conviction when making
purchasing decisions by rewarding those businesses and organizations that, in turn, support WHYY."[135]

If the St. Francis Medical System and NPR aired just one
spot providing accurate information about hysterectomy, it could
save thousands of women from surgery. That would be something
more in line with the Catholic mission of the hospital and the non-
profit radio network that calls itself a "dominant intellectual force
in American life."

Despite their rapid ascent, these surgical robots have some
serious drawbacks. A Brown University biomedical website has this
to say about robotic surgery:

> The main drawbacks to this technology are the
> steep learning curve and high cost of the de-
> vice. Though Intuitive Surgical does provide a
> training program, it took surgeons about 12-18

---

[134] http://www.npr.org/about/growth.html.
[135] http://www.whyy.org/underwriting/KnowWhoUnderwritingWHYY.html.

patients before they felt comfortable performing the procedure. One of the greatest challeng-
es facing surgeons who were training on this device was that they felt hindered by the loss of
tactile, or haptic, sensation (ability to "feel" the
tissue). The large floor-mounted patient-side
cart limits the assistant surgeon's access to the
patient.[136]

And what about the "12-18 patients" who are practiced on
by each surgeon? Does that mean teaching hospitals will now have
even higher quotas as they learn how to use these surgical robots?
The article "Suit faults training in fatal surgery" discusses the death
and subsequent lawsuit resulting from the death of a high school
teacher named Al Greenway, who underwent a Da Vinci surgery to
remove a cancerous kidney:

> A lawsuit filed Tuesday by Greenway's widow ac-
> cuses the hospital of allowing doctors inexpe-
> rienced with the robot to perform his surgery.
> The suit charges that hospital was more inter-
> ested in using its new device than in ensuring
> Greenway's safety... "It was totally unnecessary
> and avoidable death," said Tampa attorney Ste-
> ven Yerrid, who represents Brenda Greenway.
> "The conventional surgery was basically jet-
> tisoned and this robotic surgery was not only
> suggested but really pushed." ... After the sur-
> gery, Greenway began showing signs of distress,
> according to the suit. A nurse tried to find a sur-
> geon to assist in his treatment, but her request
> went unfulfilled for more than two hours, the
> suit stated... [Surgeon Tod] Fusia had attended
> a three-day certification course during which
> he did not perform a robotic organ removal,
> the lawsuit stated. After he gained certification,

[136] http://biomed.brown.edu/Courses/BI108/BI108_2005_Groups/04/davinci.html.

Fusia had performed only three robotic organ removals, according to the lawsuit... The doctor was not suspended and continued operating at the hospital, officials there said... "If you listened to that press conference, you'd think that nothing was wrong and everything was great with the robot," Yerrid said. "One Problem. The patient was dead." ...[137]

The pleasant voice-over in the St. Francis underwriting spot makes robot-assisted surgery sound graceful and holistic. You can watch a Da Vinci hysterectomy and judge for yourself. A link to a webcast of one of these surgeries is available on the St. Francis website. If you can't find it there, Da Vinci has plagued the worldwide web with such videos. As I watched a robotic surgery, the only thing I could equate it to was war—it's brutal, reckless, and dehumanizing. No matter what the surgeon's skill level is, no matter what technique he or she uses, the end result is the barbaric, unconsented removal of a woman's sex organs.

Here's the letter I wrote WHYY:
I have been a dedicated listener and supporter of NPR for many years. Although I was not pleased that NPR began accepting Corporate Sponsorship and Production Sponsorship, I understand the financial need caused by the reduction in government funding.
However, I was shocked to hear your Corporate Sponsor, St. Francis Medical System, promoting the Da Vinci surgical system for performing hysterectomy, a surgery that is damaging to women. The ethereal voice tells your listeners that this gynecologist-controlled robotic surgery is less invasive, implying that it is safe. If you watch

---

[137] Brink, Graham, "Suit Faults Training In Fatal Surgery," *St. Petersburg Times*, December 17, 2003.

the surgery being performed on the Da Vinci website (click on the video for physicians, not the sanitized public version) you will quickly see that this is a highly invasive destructive surgery. Hysterectomy is the surgical removal of the uterus, a reproductive, sexual, hormone-responsive organ that supports the bladder and bowel. Whether the surgery is performed abdominally, vaginally, laparoscopically, or by a gynecologist-controlled robot, a hormone responsive sex organ is removed, the vagina is shortened, and there is a loss of support to the bladder and bowel. Women who experienced uterine orgasm before the surgery will not experience it after the uterus is removed. When the uterus is removed women have a three times greater incidence of cardiovascular disease than women with an intact uterus, and when the ovaries are removed they have a seven times greater incidence of cardiovascular disease.

There are 22 million women in the United States whose female organs have been surgically removed. 2% were life saving and 98% were "elective," a euphemism that really means unwarranted. Girls and women are not educated about the functions of female organs, and they are not informed about the adverse effects of hysterectomy that have been well documented in medical literature for over a century.

Women who might ignore this promotion on commercial stations will be more vulnerable to it on NPR, because public radio has long been considered authoritative, idealistic and responsible in their programming. The St. Francis Health System ad that makes hysterectomy sound simple and inconsequential is dangerous to women.

NPR is no longer the station people will hear
when they are put on hold at HERS to make
sure that they will not be subjected to the Da
Vinci ad. We will not support WHYY or NPR or
listen to any of its programs until the Da Vinci
hysterectomy promotion is stopped.

Many men and women sent their own letters and emails to
WHYY and NPR.

To Talkback,
This does not seem real. A station dedicated to
honor and truth and beauty, to stoop as low as
to promote an operation that harms a woman's
body more than this, you would need to promote suicide. The Da Vinci hysterectomy, or any
hysterectomy is the biggest best kept lie in the
medical community. Doctors cover up the side
effects women have after this procedure, leave
them in pain, discredit them, and leave them
to fend for themselves afterwards, to get counseling, and medical help from the damage and
hormonal damage this operation causes. I feel
like I have been betrayed, your station is more
intelligent than to promote the castration of a
woman. Please discontinue this advertisement
with St. Francis Health System, before another
woman has her sex organs removed without being told the truth about what her options are,
clearly and concisely.Sincerely, Martha

Another HERS supporter sent a letter to WHYY, which generated this response from the radio station:

Dear Ms. Vidris:
Thank you for your e-mail and for sharing your
concerns about the St. Francis Medical System
underwriting spot currently airing on WHYY-
FM. While we appreciate your point of view
and the candor with which you express it, know
that as a public broadcasting station WHYY

accepts underwriting that complies with our FCC guidelines as stated on the WHYY Website. These can be found at http://www.whyy.org/underwriting/policy.html. The St. Francis Medical System underwriting spot complies with these guidelines. However, please be aware that broadcasting a spot on air is not an endorsement by WHYY of its underwriters, their services or products. Again, thank you for having contacted us. Although you may disagree with this particular underwriting spot, we hope that you will once again listen to WHYY.

Sincerely,
Nessa Forman
Vice President for Corporate Communications

Forman's response nagged and pulled at me. She says the ads placed on their website by the likes of Merck and Pfizer and St Francis comply with FCC regulations, but that doesn't make them okay. Where's the cut-off line of acceptability here? At what point does WHYY care more about moral outrage than FCC regulations?

We had to find out, so with a little encouragement from HERS, WHYY was flooded with more emails and letters, letting them know that many radios were falling silent until they dropped the ad. To their credit, although WHYY continued to air the ads, soon thereafter the ad was edited and no longer advertised robotic hysterectomy.

When we initiated the campaign to get public support to educate WHYY about the harmful content in their advertising, some people said, "Oh they'll never listen to you, they need the corporate money more than they need HERS listeners." My response was, "You're either part of the solution or you're part of the problem. Women are expressing their rage to HERS, and it's up to each woman to decide if they care enough to voice that outrage to NPR."

Similar things have been said about changing hysterectomy informed consent law. "Why should politicians listen to HERS when they have so much to gain from medical money?" But if you're defeated before you begin and believe that you have no power and no ability to rally support to change an injustice, then you won't.

Like NPR, politicians will respond and act when they realize that the votes that put them in their elected seats shouldn't be taken for granted. Voters will support the politician who represents the wishes and best interests of their constituency.

FORTY-TWO

Hysterectomy and the social landscape.

Albuquerque, New Mexico—Nora W. Coffey

A HERS employee told me that when he's curious about something or has an obscure question, he uses Wikipedia, the free encyclopedia that "can be edited by anyone with access to the Internet."[138] As any woman searching for information might, I went to wikipedia.com and did a search on "hysterectomy." When the entry came up I was able to read the article that anyone anywhere in the world could've posted, along with discussion from visitors and the history of all previous entries and changes to it. Predictably, the hysterectomy entry was filled with potentially harmful misinformation. So I hit the "edit" button and rewrote it. Instantaneously, accurate information about hysterectomy was available for all the world to see.

But how long was that harmful entry up there before I changed it? How many women were damaged because they landed on the old Wikipedia entry?

When I returned to Wikipedia a few days later, I found that someone had retained some of my corrections but removed others, restoring some of the previous erroneous information. This process went back and forth for a while, and I finally quit editing it because someone kept posting incorrect information after me.

By the time we arrived in Albuquerque, we had been to 40 cities in 40 states in 40 weeks. I often thought about women taking a pamphlet with them to the doctor's office, and the doctor scoffing

[138] http://en.wikipedia.org/wiki/Wikipedia:About.

at them the way the editors of the hysterectomy entry at Wikipedia brushed aside some of the facts I posted there and replaced them with myths and lies.

Because it was New Year's Day and I was tired of protesting at hospitals with no foot traffic, I decided to break our own rule and protest in front of Albuquerque Presbyterian Hospital on private property. What I was doing there couldn't have been more obvious, but after a while a woman asked, "Is this the protest?" She picked out a sign, opened her umbrella to keep the sun off her face, and stood there through most of the protest. She was shy and obviously uncomfortable protesting, but she was out there doing her part. A short while later two women arrived who had avoided surgery after being counseled by HERS.

At about 12:30, with only 30 minutes left before we were done for the day, a security guard came out of the hospital, followed by two administrators and a nurse. One of them said, "Excuse me, you're going to have to leave. This is private property, and you're not allowed to hand out information here."

I responded by handing each of them a pamphlet. I then walked away without a word. They got visibly uncomfortable, looking at each other as if to say, "Well now what do we do?"

The other protestors sat down on a bench to watch what I'd do next. This wasn't unusual—the protestors in most cities were timid when it came to exercising their rights. I resumed handing out pamphlets to everyone going in and out of the hospital.

Then one of the hospital administrators said with nervous energy, almost as an apology, "Do you know, I really think what you're doing is a good thing? But we just can't have it here."

"I understand," I said, and continued protesting.

Then the nurse came over and stood directly in front of me, reading the pamphlet I gave her. Very quietly, so no one else could hear, she echoed the other guy, saying, "I think this is a really good thing you're doing. But you have to know that you can't do it here."

"I understand," I said. "But our protest will continue." At that, the other protestors stood up and joined me again. Emboldened now, they distributed pamphlets faster than ever, frequently checking their watches. The minutes crept by, until the few remaining moments of our protest ticked away. Then we stopped, packed up our things, and left.

The next day we met at the University of New Mexico Hospital, a teaching hospital situated on a heavily trafficked street. A few of the people passing by seemed to think we were part of the abortion movement, a frequent problem wherever we went. It was understandable, because you don't often see people protesting in front of hospitals and clinics. But then there were those who seemed to go out of their way to take information from us, because they thought we *were* protesting abortion. The fact that we were both criticized and supported by both sides of the debate demonstrates that unconsented hysterectomy spans all political organizations and affiliations.

FORTY-THREE

When doctors go on strike, fewer people die.

Miami, Florida—Rick Schweikert

In his article "Iatrogenic Epidemics of Puerperal Fever in the 18th and 19th Centuries," E. Y. Bridson writes:

> The epidemics of puerperal fever…began soon after the creation of Lying-in hospitals… The primary purpose of these hospitals was to provide physicians with training in obstetrics in general and in forceps deliveries in particular.[139]

Once doctors figured out the connection between washing their hands and obstetric deaths, mortality for mother and baby plummeted. Mother and infant mortality could be greatly improved if hospitals were more sanitary, and if babies weren't delivered within the same building where infectious diseases are treated.

Gary French reports, "Hospital-acquired infections (HAIs) are common: at any one time about 1 in 10 patients in acute care hospitals have an HAI, and an additional 10-60% of infections may present after discharge."[140] Infant mortality is lower in Cuba, for example, as well as 40 other countries around the world. American hospitals may often be shiny new buildings, but hospital workers don't exercise good hygiene and hospital administrations are reluctant to invest in costly infection control. Furthermore, natural, non-interventional birthing is encouraged in Cuba and other

---

[139] Bridson, E. Y., "Iatrogenic Epidemics of Puerperal Fever in the 18th and 19th Centuries," *British Journal of Biomedical Science*, June 1996.
[140] French, Gary, *Basic Concepts of Infection Control*, Chapter 23, International Federation of Infection Control, 2007.

countries, while in America babies are frequently pulled out (forceps, vacuum, etc) or cut out (C-section) to fit the baby's delivery into the medical industry's birthing calculus, increasing the likelihood of complications and infections. About 1/3 of all babies in the U.S. are delivered during surgery. Rita Rubin of *USA Today* reports, "As the [C-section] rate has risen, so has the rate of pregnancy-associated deaths."[141]

Evaluation and treatment of most symptoms and conditions that women experience can be done by a general practitioner (GP). Although many gynecologists position themselves as primary care physicians, women would be better served by seeing a GP or an internist. It's not a good idea for women to see a surgeon for a Pap smear. Gynecology is a *surgical* subspecialty, hence the move toward surgically fertilizing women and surgically delivering babies.

In vitro fertilization (IVF) is one of the most profitable procedures for gynecologists. For all of its hype and advertising, it's important to know that IVF (surgical fertilization) is painful, invasive, expensive, and it has a 2/3 failure rate with serious risks. It can result in increased risk of ovarian cancer, ovarian hyperstimulation syndrome, multiple embryos, congenital health problems, birth defects in about 10% of IVF infants (including a three times greater risk of cerebral palsy), and death of the mother. But we're rarely told that side of the story. For more on IVF, read Gena Corea's *The Mother Machine*.[142]

---

[141]   Rubin, Rita, "Answers prove elusive as C-section rate rises," *USA Today*, January 8, 2008.
[142]   Corea, Gena, *The Mother Machine: Reproductive Technologies from Artificial Insemination to Artificial Wombs*, HarperCollins, 1985.

There's a street that runs between Miami University's medical campus and the Jackson Memorial Hospital. It's named for Georgios N. Papanicolaou, the inventor of the Pap smear. The Pap smear is often praised as a medical miracle because it's sometimes effective in detecting cervical cancer, but it is prone to a high percentage of errors. One report puts the error rate of false-positive results (tests that say a woman has cancer but she doesn't) at 44.8%.[143] Other studies indicate an even higher percentage rate of false-negative results (when a test tells a woman she doesn't have cancer, but she does).[144] Because of the high error rate, women with abnormal Pap smears might find the results more meaningful if they repeat the test three times.

The natural condition of the cervix is to have some degree of inflammation. Chronic cervicitis is so common it can be called the natural state of the cervix and often results in abnormal Pap smears. Women who use hot tubs or whirlpools (breeding grounds for spreading genital viruses, even among family members), don't use a condom, or who are sexually active are much more vulnerable to developing cervical dysplasia or a genital virus.

Cervical dysplasia is an appearance of abnormal cells on the cervix, and can in some rare instances be a precursor to cervical cancer. Most cervical dysplasia is caused by human papilloma virus (HPV). There are over a hundred types of HPV, but only a few have a high malignant potential. A Polymerase Chain Reaction test narrows the range of the particular type of virus causing

[143]   Hoekstra AV, Kosinski A, Huh WK, "Hormonal contraception and false-positive cervical cytology: is there an association?" *Journal of Lower Genital Tract Disease*, April 2006.
[144]   Ku, NN, "Automated Papanicolaou smear analysis as a screening tool for female lower genital tract malignancies," *Current Opinion in Obstetrics & Gynecology*, February 1999.

the dysplasia. If dysplasia is found, most gynecologists recommend colposcopy (a scope used to look at the cervix) and a "punch biopsy" (similar to a paper punch, tissue is removed and sent to a lab for microscopic exam). If early cervical cancer is detected, it may be treatable by removing the affected tissue with a wire loop called a LEEP procedure.

But with about 11,000 cases of cervical cancer detected each year in the U.S. (1/10th of 1% of the female population) it's only slightly more prevalent than the incidence of testicular and penile cancer.[145] Also, do-it-herself Pap smear tests have been around for years, and several websites provide testimony from women who find it works well for them.[146]

Despite some treatment successes, it isn't at all clear whether more doctors are good for our health. In fact, the opposite may be true. John Bunker presented the following in his article "The Role Of Medical Care In Contributing To Health Improvements Within Societies":

> Treatment can shorten as well as lengthen life expectancy. This is dramatically evident in surgery and anaesthesia which, however well performed, entail some risk of death and has been used to explain, at least in part, differences in life expectancy between countries. The two-fold greater rates of discretionary surgery in America, relative to England and Wales, that I reported in 1970 could thus be expected to reflect this risk and was estimated to account for a third to a half of the greater life expectancy in England and Wales at that time…

---

[145] Centers for Disease Control and Prevention (CDC), National Center for Health Statistics (NCHS).

[146] Fournier Self Sampling Cervical Test; Sen-C-Test.

Iatrogenic [medical error] mortality may similarly help to explain the observations by Cochrane and by Carr-Hill and their associates that greater numbers of doctors and medical resources, and presumably more discretionary medical and surgical care, are associated with higher death rates. Iatrogenic mortality is also reflected in the observation of brief but dramatic decreases in population death rate when doctors strike and surgery for elective (but not emergency) operations are suspended.[147]

More doctors and more procedures equals higher death rates. An article titled "Doctors' Strike In Israel May Be Good For Health" suggests that doctor strikes result in decreased mortality:

"The number of funerals we have performed has fallen drastically," said Hananya Shahor, the veteran director of Jerusalem's Kehilat Yerushalayim burial society. "This month, there were only 93 funerals compared with 153 in May 1999, 133 in the same month in 1998, and 139 in May 1997,' he said. The society handles 55% of all deaths in the Jerusalem metropolitan area. Last April, there were only 130 deaths compared with 150 or more in previous Aprils. "I can't explain why," said Mr Shahor. Meir Adler, manager of the Shamgar Funeral Parlour, which buries most other residents of Jerusalem, declared with much more certainty: "There definitely is a connection between the doctors' sanctions and fewer deaths. We saw the same thing in 1983" [when the Israel Medical Association applied sanctions for four and a half months].[148]

---

[147]   Bunker, John P., "The Role Of Medical Care In Contributing To Health Improvements Within Societies," *International Journal of Epidemiology*, 2001.
[148]   Siegel-Itzkovich, Judy, "Doctors' Strike In Israel May Be Good For Health," *British Medical Journal*, June 2000.

The same was true during a Los Angeles County doctors strike. And when 20,000 doctors in Germany went on strike. And during a doctor strike in England. And during a two-month work stoppage by doctors in Bogata. The result: mortality decreased.

There are many frightening newspaper, medical journal, and online articles written on the subject. "When Doctors Strike, Fewer People Die" by Jurriaan Kamp is particularly telling.[149] Kamp rejects the claim that modern medicine is responsible for increased longevity. Instead, he credits Thomas Crapper as "one of humanity's greatest benefactors" for inventing the common toilet. Kamp says that because of the toilet and sewage treatment, "Cholera, typhoid, tuberculosis, and dysentery were already on the decline when antibiotics and vaccines were introduced." Not only have many vaccinations not been proven to be effective, many have been proven to be very harmful. As homebirth advocate Dr. Mayer Eisenstein said, "Children that aren't vaccinated never get Autism."[150] Kamp rightly refers to emergency care, not vaccinations or Pap smears or surgeries or drugs, as the greatest advance in modern medicine, claiming that aside from emergent care the industrial medical establishment has "sadly little to offer."[151]

---

[149] Kamp, Jurriaan, "When Doctors Strike, Fewer People Die," *Ode Magazine*, and http://www.geocities.com/missionstmichael/Doctors.html.

[150] Cristian, Arthur, "Children That Aren't Vaccinated Never Get Autism!" *UPI*, December 7, 2005.

[151] For more on vaccines: Stevenson, Heidi, "Dissecting a Thimerosal Study," *NaturalNews.com*, November 14, 2007 and Stevenson, Heidi "Childhood Vaccinations Hoax - Not Effective and at Worst, Harmful," *NaturalNews.com*, February 08, 2008. In 1979, Sweden banned the pertussis (whooping cough) vaccine given to American infants, for example, and now Sweden has the second lowest infant mortality rate in the world, whereas the U.S. comes in at a miserable 42nd, according to the CIA's "World Fact Book," https://www.cia.gov/library/publications/the-world-factbook/rankorder/2091rank.html.

Two theater companies answered our request for proposals to host readings of *un becoming* in Miami. The first was Fantasy Theater's reading on Friday night before the first day of the protest, directed by Faride Jamin and staged at St. John's Church in Miami Beach on a patio that looked out onto Surprise Lake. A young woman with exquisitely braided hair quietly wept during the reading. Another nursed her baby in the back of the audience to keep the baby from crying.

Some of the audience joined us the next morning at the protest. Two of them, Ted and Ernie, were vigorous supporters. They moved to Florida from New Jersey after Ted retired as a police officer. Ernie was a student nurse who called HERS to get information about her fibroids and urinary stress incontinence.

Urinary stress incontinence is leakage caused by pressure to the bladder occurring during coughing, sneezing, and physical activity. According to the American Urogynecologic Society, "Involuntary loss of urine is reportedly experienced by upwards of 95% of women in their reproductive and post-menopausal years."[152] Ernie had the symptoms of a slight cystocele (sagging bladder), so HERS sent her some exercises that usually help considerably (see the New Jersey chapter).

Although her fibroids were asymptomatic, meaning they were present but with no negative symptoms, the doctor told Ernie she needed a hysterectomy. "At the very least," he said, "I need get in there and take a look around." So she agreed to exploratory surgery. "But that's all I agreed to," Ernie said, "and I told him I definitely didn't want a hysterectomy."

---

[152] "Bladder Control Problems," *American Urogynecologic Society*, http://www. mypelvichealth.org/WhatarePelvicFloorDisorders/BladderControlProblems/tabid/85/ Default.aspx.

Ernie knew something wasn't right the minute she woke up from surgery. She tried to convince her family she'd be okay, but she often wept and screamed uncontrollably and fell into sudden fits of rage. Her life came to a crashing halt. She needed answers to why she felt so sad and enraged.

It wasn't until a week after the exploratory surgery that Ernie was told that the doctor had hysterectomized her. And then two weeks later Ernie received the bill from the hospital. In the list of charges were the letters: BSO—bilateral salpingo-oophorectomy (removal of both ovaries and fallopian tubes). The doctor left her to figure out when she received the hospital bill that he had also removed her ovaries. "While he was in there," Ernie said, "he castrated me."

She called HERS and described to Nora the gruesome, disfiguring scar the doctor left on her belly. Doctors often refer to the position of the cut as a "bikini-line incision"—a horizontal cut just above the pubic hairline, also called a Pfannensteil incision. It's something most women are unconcerned about, but it's subliminal programming. The real message is that the surgery won't be a big deal because the scar won't be visible. But after the surgery, the type of incision the doctor made was the least of Ernie's worries. Even still, the scar that Ernie described was more disfiguring than most. The doctor made an unusual vertical incision, leaving a grotesque scar with a hook on the end.

To Ernie, the scar was a visible reminder that she'd never be her old self again. Nora said, "I know what you want to hear, but I won't lie to you. You've heard enough lies from doctors. What you really want is to have your female organs back so you can be who you were before the surgery. I wish I could tell you what you want to hear, but hysterectomy can only be done—it can't be undone."

In spite of her problems, Ernie said it was a "great relief" to find HERS. Nora put her in touch with other women in her area HERS had counseled, and Nora recommended an attorney to file a malpractice lawsuit. She also helped Ernie prepare for the deposition and invited her to the HERS conference that year in Philadelphia.

At the conference her husband Ted figured women would be uncomfortable with a man there, so he sat alone in the last row. Ernie cried through the entire conference and didn't say anything until the wrap-up, when women usually begin to feel comfortable speaking about their own experiences. After a few other women spoke, Ernie stood with tears streaming down her face, trembling with anger as she described what had been done to her.

Ernie and Ted have attended many HERS conferences since then, and each time they speak a little more freely. Ted tells how Ernie's rage was directed at him because he was a safe target for her anger. He'd come home from work and Ernie would be pacing from wall to wall. With such raw emotion and anguish, anything he said brought on a physical assault from Ernie, who scratched his chest and face.

"I just didn't think there was any way I could live the rest of my life this way," Ernie told me. But no one knows how much they can endure until they're forced to live with much more than they ever thought was possible.

We set up our protest at one of the entrances to the Jackson Memorial Hospital. From the protest site we could see a sign on a pedestrian overpass that said "Papanicolaou Way." There was a small park at the beginning of the long driveway leading into the medical center campus. Two men sat in a van parked in the first spot of the parking lot closest to the driveway entrance, with the motor running. They watched our every move. In the driveway, there were six police squad cars lined up. Even with all we'd been through, it was a little intimidating, which of course was their goal.

A steady flow of cars rolled down their windows to take a pamphlet as they waited at the light. Every 15 minutes or so transit riders arrived and departed on city buses and the Metrorail. Many asked us, "Are those cops here for you?"

Just then I noticed an elderly couple crest the hill at the top of the driveway behind the police cars. The man trailed a few steps behind, and the woman had a large sign tied around her neck with handwritten words I couldn't make out at first. As they approached, I called Nora over to have a look.

Dorothy and her husband Dolph had parked in one of the hospital garages. It was a sweltering day and Dolph, recuperating from hip and knee substitute surgery, struggled to keep up. He veered away from Dorothy and headed for the park benches in the shade.

We were careful to stay off hospital property with all those cops around, but there was Dorothy marching down the hill past them with a 3' by 2' poster board tied around her neck. On the sign in magic marker was a list of all of the problems hysterectomy had caused her. I was proud when she marched past the line of police cars and joined our ranks. "That's right," I thought, "she's with us."

I was prepared for the worst, expecting the police to get out of their cars and harass Dorothy, but she was oblivious to them. She said hello to us, picked up some pamphlets, and began distributing information as if it was something she did every day. We continued distributing information until 1:00 p.m. as usual, before packing up and calling it a day.

The second Miami reading of *un becoming* was held in the Wertheim Performing Arts Center at Florida International University. Directed by drama professor Jeffrey Tangeman, his student actors did a really superb job. In the talkback the mother of one of the actors told the audience she was especially pleased to see her daughter in the performance, because she herself had been hysterectomized. Her husband, the actor's father, was very vocal about the impact of unwarranted surgeries on families and communities.

Someone asked. "When is a hysterectomy necessary?"

"A hysterectomy is never necessary," Nora said, "because 'necessary' means it's required…that you have no choice. But you always have a choice. If you have uterine cancer or ovarian cancer that has spread beyond those organs, no amount of surgery or chemotherapy will save you, as was portrayed in Margaret Edson's play *Wit*. There are a few instances—about 2% of all hysterectomies—in which the surgery itself might save your life, but it's always your option to choose no treatment."

FORTY-FOUR

Under the guise of exploratory surgery.

Nashville, Tennessee—Nora W. Coffey

> Physicians and politicians resemble one another
> in this respect: some defend the constitution,
> and others destroy it. —Author unknown

The most powerful seat in Congress is the Senate Majority Leader, which for a time was occupied by Bill Frist of Tennessee. Visitors to his website were greeted with the former senator's title of choice, "Bill Frist, M.D." Frist cultivated an image as *the good doctor* throughout his political career, but Doug Ireland of the *LA Weekly News* called him "the Bad Doctor" and referred to his years in politics as a "long record of corporate vices."[153]

Frist's family rose to prominence by building up HCA, the largest for-profit hospital chain in the country. Andrew Ross Sorkin reports that the nation's largest non-profit hospital chain was sold to "three private-equity firms and the family of Senator Bill Frist, the Senate majority leader, whose father, the late Dr. Thomas Frist Sr., and his brother, Dr. Thomas F. Frist Jr., founded HCA."[154] At the time of this writing, HCA is the nation's largest for-profit hospital chain. Frist is emblematic of the cozy relationship between medicine and politics, and how corporate medicine has managed to infiltrate and co-opt the democratic process.

---

[153] Ireland, Doug, "The Bad Doctor—Bill Frist's long record of corporate vices," *LA Weekly News*, January 9, 2003.
[154] Sorkin, Andrew Ross, "HCA Buyout Highlights Era of Going Private," *New York Times*, July 25, 2006.

John Nichols suggests that Frist's "primary purpose in the Senate [was] enriching his already wealthy family."

> The wealthy doctor ran for the Senate in 1994 with a simple mission: to prevent health care reforms that might pose a threat to his family's stake in Columbia/HCA, the nation's leading owner of hospitals... By blocking needed health care reforms, pushing for tort reforms that would limit malpractice payouts and supporting moves to privatize Medicare, Frist pumped up his family's fortunes at the expense of Americans who lacked access to health care.[155]

Robert Dreyfuss writes in *Mother Jones*:

> This senator handles his family company's legislative prescriptions... Some companies hire lobbyists to work Congress. Some have their executives lobby directly. But Tennessee's Frist family, the founders of Columbia/HCA Healthcare Corp., the nation's largest hospital conglomerate, has taken it a step further: They sent an heir to the Senate. And there, with disturbingly little controversy, Republican Sen. Bill Frist has co-sponsored bills that may allow his family's company to profit from the ongoing privatization of Medicare. The senator's father, Dr. Thomas Frist Sr., was a founder of Columbia/HCA, the country's biggest chain of for-profit hospitals, a $20 billion health care empire that includes 340 hospitals, 135 outpatient surgery centers, and 200 home health care agencies in 38 states. The family has spent lavishly on political campaigns for years.[156]

[155] Nichols, John, "Farewell to Senator Bill Frist, R-Frist Family" *The Nation*, November 29, 2006.

[156] Dreyfuss, Robert, "Frist Aid," *Mother Jones*, May 1, 1997.

And Bill Theobald with Gannett reports "Hastert, Frist Said to Rig Bill for Drug Firms":

> Senate Majority Leader Bill Frist and House Speaker Dennis Hastert engineered a backroom legislative maneuver to protect pharmaceutical companies from lawsuits, say witnesses to the pre-Christmas power play. The language was tucked into a Defense Department appropriations bill at the last minute without the approval of members of a House-Senate conference committee, say several witnesses, including a top Republican staff member.[157]

"It sucks," one of Frist's colleagues said of the law. "That was an absolute travesty," said another. Another called it "an insult to the legislative process."

The evidence demonstrates that Frist was little more than a lobbyist in a powerful political office. Even a spate of HCA criminal penalties mounting into the billions of dollars seemed little more than minor inconveniences to the politician who presented himself as a pious Presbyterian leading a political party that was partly swept into power by touting Christian values. HCA criminal penalties were merely another deal to be negotiated:

> Combined with previous settlements HCA has negotiated with the government involving fraud accusations—including its agreement in 2000 to plead guilty to 14 felonies—the company will be paying a total of more than $1.7 billion in civil and criminal penalties, by far the largest amount ever secured by federal prosecutors in a health care fraud case.[158]

[157] Theobald, Bill, "Hastert, Frist Said to Rig Bill for Drug Firms," *The Gannett News Service*, February 9, 2006.
[158] Eichenwald, Kurt, "HCA Is Said To Reach Deal On Settlement Of Fraud Case," *New York Times*, December 18, 2002.

Consider that the next time you're in the Music City driving down Broadway past the Frist Center For The Visual Arts. What a gift to the people of middle Tennessee, this wonderful museum in Nashville, but what a price taxpayers and visitors to Frist hospitals had to pay to make these benefactors rich enough to endow it. It required a few generations of Frists lapping at the legislative trough and defrauding American taxpayers out of Medicare dollars.

And what does Bill Frist have to say about healthcare reform? The following statement regarding medical malpractice "reform" is from Frist's official government website and sums up his position:

> Again and again we hear the horror stories - trauma centers closing, doctors striking, specialists quitting, and expectant mothers having serious difficulty even finding a doctor. The President is right. This is a crisis of health care access and skyrocketing costs, and we know what needs to done - passing meaningful medical litigation reform. I don't want this issue to be slowed by petty politics. We must act soon before the quality of health care is further compromised...[159]

The only medical litigation reform we need is to *increase* the public's ability to sue companies like HCA for wrongdoing, to hold their doctors and administrators accountable. The worst horror stories (to use Frist's own words) that I know of regarding Medicare are the ones where companies like HCA bilked taxpayers out of mountains of hard-earned money that could be used to help Tennesseans get emergency healthcare. It seems to me that one of the quickest ways to reform Medicaid/Medicare and the health-

---

[159] Frist, Bill, "Comments On Medical Malpractice Reform," January 16, 2003.

care system is to deny the Frists and corporations like HCA access to the legislative troughs that make them rich at the expense of the rest of us. The robber barons of yore never left us—they simply moved from selling steel and railroads to medicine.

But Frist and Columbia/HCA aren't alone. Entering "politicians influenced by drug companies" into an internet search engine reveals more accounts of corporate medicine interference with legislation than you'll ever care to read. The Frists didn't invent this powerful manipulation of politics and medicine. They just mastered it, upped the ante, and then used their influence to support self-serving interests. The record $1.7 billion in settlements Columbia/HCA agreed to pay out was the result of a ten-year investigation, paid for by taxpayers. No one was arrested. Two were convicted, but both were acquitted on appeals. Perhaps worst of all, Columbia/HCA was allowed access to Medicare funds in the future, so there's nothing preventing them from defrauding us of our tax dollars again.

The Frists and HCA aren't the only ones making a mint manipulating our country's medical system. Milt Freundenheim reports, "The pharmaceutical industry is beginning to reap a windfall from a surprisingly lucrative niche market: drugs for poor people."[160] The pharmaceutical industry has long been known for its insipid system of gift-giving and freebies to doctors, nurses, and medical staffs, with the expectation that their products will be touted to their patients. The American Medical Student Association's (AMSA) PharmFree Initiative encourages medical students to "pledge to accept no money, gifts, or hospitality from the pharma-

---

[160] Freundenheim, Milt, "A Windfall From Shifts to Medicare," *New York Times*, July 17, 2006.

ceutical industry; to seek unbiased sources of information and not rely on information disseminated by drug companies; and to avoid conflicts of interest in medical education and practice." Here's an email received from a medical student on a listserv I belong to:

Date: Wed, 30 Nov 2005 18:22:44 -0500
To: AMSA Primary Care
Subject: [primary] PharmFree - free pens vs. morals/ethics
A good evening to everyone,
Given that today is AMSA's PharmFree day, I thought I would write in hopes of instigating some conversation, personal reflection, and action on the issue of the pharmaceutical industry's infiltration into every last nook and cranny of medicine.
It is truly sickening (and depressing) to me to see the way we have sold out as a profession to the drug companies...we write with their pens, take notes on their paper, eat their food, tell time by their clocks, staple with their staplers... pitiful!
I am in a primary care setting where I see the drug reps set up lunch everyday for the entire office, right in the only lunchroom there is... and the entire medical staff flocks to their food, their freebies, and the "enlightening conversation" that the reps will provide. (Interestingly, one physician in this practice who came from a nearby low-income clinic says that she saw a total of 1 pharm rep. come to that clinic in her 4 years there...I wonder why!)
How can medicine, a field based on the simple ethical principle that we are here to do what is best for our patients have made such "bosom buddy" connections with an industry whose simple underlying principle is to profit off the sale of their products to our patients (which

obviates the need to sweet talk the people taking care of those patients—US!)???????

My friends, as I have started to read what literature there is out there, a few things are blatantly obvious:

1) Physicians consistently underestimate the extent to which they are influenced in their prescribing behaviors by pharm. reps and the larger pharm. industry

2) There is NO evidence to support the idea that maintaining close ties with the drug reps. reduces the cost that your patients pay out of pocket for medicines...yes, there may be a few samples given of an expensive new drug which has no efficacy data superior to an older generic, and then when it comes time for refills, guess who is now going to pay a lot more than they would have otherwise?

3) The drug industry is not stupid - the fact that there has been a 40% increase in drug reps over recent years and the fact that the industry puts 13 billion dollars annually into advertising directly to physicians should tell us something about the assumption amongst physicians that "we are not influenced by the drug companies"

So, let us, the next wave of physicians, begin to take seriously our ethical/moral duty (to do what is best for our patients) and stop taking lunches, pens and whatever other junk is thrown at us...start reading, educating others, and begin discussing with physicians that you work with these issues!

Educate yourself:

AMSA's stance http://www.amsa.org/prof/history.cfm

NO FREE LUNCH http://www.nofreelunch.org/

It was a bitterly cold January morning in Nashville, and we had a protest to get underway. In spite of the cold, I met with two protestors, Julia and John, at the Baptist Hospital (yet another institution named after a saint), which is under the corporate umbrella of the Saint Thomas Health Services and Ascension Health, the largest not-for-profit healthcare system in the United States.

Even before we arrived at Baptist we had work to do. Our protest materials hadn't arrived from New Mexico. But John, who was a science professor at Vanderbilt University, didn't miss a beat. We hopped back into their car and drove to his office to make new signs and pamphlets. Julia waited in the car as John and I went into his office in Vanderbilt's Stevenson Center.

As we walked through Stevenson, John gave me a tour of the stunning yellow tile floor that Julia had designed and the magnificent paintings she completed before her hysterectomy. Having seen some of Julia's artwork before the surgery, I was curious how her work might've changed after. When I asked John, he said, "I think you'd better ask Julia about that."

Within minutes of arriving in one of the classrooms, John recreated protest signs that were identical to the ones that didn't arrive from New Mexico. We returned to Julia and drove to a copy store. Along with the missing signs, we had no pamphlets, but I usually kept a few with me. So we printed a few hundred pamphlets to hand out until more materials could be overnighted from HERS. In less than of hour of meeting John and Julia, we were back in business, setting up our protest.

John was a quick study. He watched me hand a pamphlet to a woman through her car window, and he immediately ran down an entire line of cars, passing pamphlets out to each one of them. Whatever he said to them it was working, because almost everyone took a pamphlet. When they didn't take one, John simply moved on to the next car. But when this happened to Julia, it was obvious that she felt personally rejected.

I'd seen this happen before. Protesting was much more personal for hysterectomized women than their families. Julia was a very private person, and she was still grappling with being public about what had been done to her. When someone refused to take a pamphlet, it represented the denial of her own experiences. Or worse, it was a reminder that some people don't care about what's being done to women.

Julia didn't have to encounter much rejection, though, because almost everyone in Nashville was receptive to our message and took information from us. They might have been more receptive because we were out there in such abominable weather. We got similar responses in other protest locations where people were appreciative that someone cared enough to protest in conditions that deterred most people from being out there for pleasure, let alone educating the public.

After packing up for the day, we went to a deli for lunch. I ordered, then John ordered next, but Julia said, "Nothing for me, thank you." It seemed a little odd, but I didn't want to make her feel awkward by asking about it. When our food came Julia took a small container out of her bag, saying, "I can't eat in restaurants."

There are some aftereffects that all women experience after their female organs are removed—they're a matter of anatomical fact. But because the endocrine system is so complex and we're all wired a little differently, other aftereffects vary from woman to woman. After Julia's surgery she developed an intolerance to many kinds of food (especially "prepared" or "processed" foods), and she's extremely sensitive to many chemicals. Julia couldn't come into the Stevenson Center to print protest signs with us because it was filled with labs that used chemicals. And she would've gotten sick eating the food John and I ordered.

That night I accepted an invitation to have dinner at their home. Their house stood in a wooded lot at the foot of a steep, rocky hill. From the outside it was a simple, rectangular, ordinary home. But when the front door opened I entered a stunning foyer with one-of-a-kind furniture, paintings, and sculpture everywhere.

Julia prepared a few simple dishes for herself as we enjoyed her gourmet cooking. As I complimented her on dinner, John said, "She's the Beethoven of cooking. She can't taste her own creations anymore, but that doesn't stop her from creating masterpieces."

Of all of the works of art in their home, there was one in particular that really captivated me. It depicted a long, winding blue wall that snaked off into the distance. As I got closer, I realized that the wall was comprised of intertwined bodies with a sort of Escher influence. Each one of the hundreds and hundreds of bodies in the painting was distinct and unique in detail, but they blended together so gracefully that with a quick glance it appeared to be nothing more than a wall twisting and turning through the countryside. I asked myself, 'Am I looking at a painting she did before or after the surgery?'

When we sat down with an after-dinner drink, I asked, "Are your paintings for sale?"

"I guess so," she said. "I haven't really thought about it much."

"If I could have any of them," I said cautiously, "I'd buy the one with the wall of people."

"Oh no, you can't have that one," she replied with a laugh. "That's John's favorite."

Most women I meet are eager to talk with me about their experiences with hysterectomy. But Julia was different. She was reserved. And then suddenly there it was, we were talking about it. I felt that pain of empathy as the horrible suspense of her all-too-familiar story unfolded.

Julia made it clear to the gynecologist that she didn't want surgery of any kind. Still, the doctor convinced her to undergo "exploratory" surgery "just to take a look around."

John was in the waiting room, and the surgeon came out to speak with him during the surgery. He told John that Julia's "condition" was far worse than was previously thought. The doctor implied that Julia could die if he didn't remove her uterus and ovaries immediately. This, it turned out, was a flat out lie.

Often, spouses and parents in this situation harbor a lot of anger, hurt, and grief that they allowed a doctor permission to do this to their wife or daughter. Some couples can't stay together afterwards. With other couples like Julia and John, there's an understanding of the terrible decision the doctor foisted on John. In that moment of urgency, John believed that by signing the consent form he was doing what he needed to save Julia's life.

Julia continued going back to the doctor, telling him she wasn't at all well since the surgery. Most days it was all she could do to get out of bed. Meanwhile, Julia got sick every time she ate, and every chemical she touched or smelled made her ill. Many women develop allergies post-hysterectomy they didn't have before, but Julia appeared to be allergic to everything she ate, touched, or breathed. The doctors were clueless, but she continued to search for answers, finally discovering a doctor in Texas who founded an institute focused on allergies. She spent a lot of time there in a controlled environment until her health finally improved a little.

Soon she was able to function enough to return home, but her life would never be the same again.

Thanks to John and Julia, Nashville was one of my most enjoyable and memorable cities of the tour. Largely because of them, we held HERS 25th Hysterectomy Conference in Nashville with a screening of the *un becoming* DVD at the legendary Belcourt Theatre.

As the plane taking me home to Philly lifted up off the runway, I felt strongly that with amazing people like Julia and John standing shoulder to shoulder with us, we were one giant step closer to stopping this from being done to another generation of women.

FORTY-FIVE

Hysterectomy and suicide.

Las Vegas, Nevada—Nora W. Coffey

Judy, our contact person in Las Vegas, met the doctor who operated on her about an hour *after* he hysterectomized her. The only "problems" she experienced before the surgery were common menstrual cramps and mood swings. She was told hysterectomy would cure both, but Judy said, "I'd do anything to have my life back."

We were interviewed together in the local newspaper. As I told the reporter and photographer about the things women consistently report after hysterectomy, the photographer stood there stunned. He then told us about some of the problems women in his family were having since the surgery.

Many young people around the country told us about a favorite aunt who was once very social, throwing big parties and planning family outings. But after the surgery she stopped entertaining, and her family couldn't get her out of the house. One young woman in Las Vegas said, "I used to do stuff with my grandmama all the time, but she had *that*," referring to the H word on the sign I was holding. "Then she always canceled on me last minute. I just stopped asking her to do stuff. Do you think that has anything to do with this?"

Before Judy's surgery she did a lot of physical labor and body building. As she said, "I used to take great pride in my body." But now she couldn't exercise at all. "It hurts too much to even do the smallest things," she said. She tried swimming, but even the seam of her suit against her skin was painful.

Then there was Judy's surgical scar. She described it as, "the worst scar I've ever seen." The doctor told her there was nothing unusual about it, but Judy sent me the before and after photos.

The first photo was of Judy with her daughter and husband on a boat. She wore a bikini—not an ounce of fat, her muscles as toned as a professional athlete. In the second photo Judy was alone in her bedroom with a horrible, mutilating scar across her belly. It looked like a big fishing hook with a flap of loose skin hanging over it. The scar was still bruised a year later, and it was indented in some places and bulged up above the surface of the skin in other places. In part because of this deformity, Judy now never let her husband see her naked.

Doctors refer to them as "apron scars" because the skin above the incision drapes over it in folds. It's common enough for it to have its own name, and it's common enough that hundreds of women have described their scars that way to me.

A few doctors recommended cosmetic surgery, but she couldn't afford it. She wasn't able to return to work, and her husband now struggled to cover the bills. She couldn't get legal representation because she "consented" to the surgery. Commit a crime with a gun, and you go to prison. Commit a crime with a scalpel, and you get rich.

It's no coincidence that 75.2% of women report a loss of sexual desire and almost the exact same percentage, 76.9%, experience profound fatigue following hysterectomy. Each statistic from the HERS Adverse Effects Data relates to all the others.[161] When the uterus is removed, sexual energy is lost. The more sexual and sensual a woman is, the more she has to lose. But these

[161] "Adverse Effects Data," HERS Foundation, www.hersfoundation.org/effects.html.

statistics are nothing new. In 1973, findings published in *The Lancet* said 70% of women experience persistent, extreme fatigue and profound depression post-hysterectomy.[162]

Most women aren't aware that the painful uterine contractions they experience during labor are produced by the same muscles that create the pleasurable contractions during uterine orgasm. There's no way to identify where the sensation of orgasm emanates from, until the uterus is removed.

The uterus is the center, the core of a woman. It's no surprise that its removal affects women in so many ways. One of the many early realizations I had of the literal centering effect of my uterus was while swimming. Growing up a bicycle ride from the ocean, swimming was part of my everyday life. I've always enjoyed floating with my arms outstretched. It required no effort, my buoyant body gracefully balanced on the surface of the water. But after the surgery, my body rolled to the right. It required constant effort to not roll to one side.

I had more sexual energy and vitality than most people I knew. What I didn't know until it was taken was how much my uterus had to do with it. The connection between sexual energy and overall vitality is well known and talked about in men. Especially in politicians, soldiers, and athletes—sexual prowess is worn as a badge. But not so for women. For women to acknowledge their sexual prowess in many ways remains taboo. I had no idea my sexuality and sensuality could be taken from me.

I can still send signals to a man if I choose to, but it surprises me when men respond. It leaves me feeling odd and a bit deceptive, like I should say, "Don't you see I'm not the woman I

---

[162] Richards, D. H., "Depression Following Hysterectomy," *The Lancet*, 1973.

once was?" When flirting is intellectual, it requires a conscious effort. That effort soon becomes tedious, whereas before it was spontaneous and exhilarating. Occasionally I feel like I should try to do something "normal" like be with a man socially. But although I can arouse it in them, it barely interests me. I'm not even a glimmer of the highly sexual person I once was.

My longtime colleague and close friend Joanne was opposed to publishing the Adverse Effects Data on the HERS website. She didn't want women's experiences to be seen as numbers, figures on a page representing a woman, a person, a life. If we were to publish them, she said, we should put them into a context that would explain the impact on each individual woman, each individual life, and the impact on society as a whole.

There's no doubt she was right—it would've been better to put the statistics in the larger, more personal context of how and why hysterectomy and castration ruins lives. That's the purpose of this book, to demonstrate woman by woman, city by city, state by state the inside-story of hysterectomy in this country. But countless women have been empowered to say no to hysterectomy after reading the Adverse Effects Data statistics on the HERS website. And countless others have had their hysterectomy experiences validated there for the first time.

Protesting in front of the University of Nevada-Las Vegas Medical Center, a car pulled over but wasn't able to stop quickly enough. The driver veered into a nearby parking lot and circled around. She stayed in the car, so I walked over to her. "I need to talk with you!" she said.

I thought she was angry, but after the usual, "What's this all about?" she calmed down a little. She spoke quickly about being hysterectomized a couple of years before and now had so many problems she wasn't able to work. Her husband grew impatient for her to return to her old self, and finally they separated. She had a child, so she had no choice but to move in with her father. It embarrassed her, she said, because she wasn't capable of being independent. She told me all of this in a deliberate, straightforward way, intent on getting the facts right.

She'd been denied disability and was "flat broke," but she insisted on giving us something. She dumped the contents of her purse onto the passenger seat and scooped up all the money she had—a handful of coins. When I hesitated, she said, "Here, take it! I know it's not much. Please?" I opened my hand and took the coins. I knew it was symbolic more than anything else. She needed to give what she could.

"I'd come back tomorrow," she said, "but they're repossessing my car." Everything else—her furniture, her home—had already been taken away. She said she'd try to figure out a way to get back to the protest, but she didn't know how. We never saw her again.

Each woman finds her own way of living with the aftermath. Some women can't confront it and need to deny it even to themselves, to function the best they can in their daily lives. For other women it's an awareness that slowly dawns on them while attending a HERS conference or visiting our website. And for women like my friend Genevieve Carmanati, the realization was immediate. "I was always aware of my uterus, like I was aware of my heartbeat," Genny once wrote. "I felt the loss of it immediately. There was a centering that was gone."

Most women come out of the operating room not knowing that the profound changes they're experiencing are permanent. Except for the scar when the surgery is abdominal or laparoscopic, there's no outward physical sign to explain what they're feeling. They know something has changed, but they're terrified to dwell on it. Disbelief and denial let them believe that someday, somehow they'll wake up and it'll all have been a bad dream. They need to not let that living nightmare enter their conscious thoughts, but it never goes away.

Every morning millions of hysterectomized women wake up and know before their feet hit the floor what kind of a day they're going to have. If their legs feel like lead, they're going to have a difficult day. If they're having trouble focusing and thinking, it's going to be an exasperating day of trying to remember common words and names. If they feel focused when they wake up, they might function fairly well. Throughout the day, they think things they never thought before, because their bodies don't act in a spontaneous way like they once did.

They convince themselves they're just tired, which they are. Maybe they never had a problem sleeping before, but now they have insomnia. If they're lucky they might fall back asleep, but often that's all the sleep they're going to get. When they can sleep it's not the deep REM sleep that once refreshed them. It's a lighter, superficial, shorter sleep. Many women stop dreaming altogether within the first year after surgery. Those who do dream say it's different, not like the realistic dreams they used to have.

Because they've never heard anyone talk about any of this, they think they must be losing their minds. To stop the dark thoughts from invading and dominating their consciousness, many women keep a television or radio on at all times, so the white noise will stave off dwelling on the physical and emotional pain.

In the shower, hair falls out in their hands in clumps. Clothes don't fit the same way anymore—they're the same size on top, but two sizes larger on the bottom. They walk differently. Each leg feels like it weighs a ton. That natural sway in their hips is gone. Even tactile sensations are different. When someone touches them, it's dull, like there's something between them and the other person—not even their skin feels like it's theirs anymore. At first they pull away when someone initiates contact, because what felt good before is now irritating. But soon they realize the impact that not wanting to be touched has on all of their relationships.

Many women have told me the doctor suggested they go buy some sexy lingerie to spice up their relationship with their husband. It's like telling a soldier with an amputated leg he should go out and buy a pair of dancing shoes to cheer himself up.

It all sounds too unbelievable to be true, so who can they talk with about it? Not even their closest friends would understand. What would they say? "I went into an operating room as the person you've known all these years and I saw in the mirror each morning, but I came out someone else, a different person." It sounds bizarre. Who can you say that to, without the other person thinking you've lost your mind? If it scares women to admit that to themselves, it's bound to scare anyone you tell it to.

Many women say, "One day I have this horrible pain in my side I can't quite put my finger on, and then it's gone for a day or two before it returns." Everything becomes unpredictable. "I'll meet you later" becomes "*maybe* I'll meet you later," because you know you might not be physically or emotionally able to meet any-one. Women never really get used to the stranger who has replaced them. You think you're handling it just fine, but then you move the wrong way and there it is.

Imagine for a moment that you're one of those women who holds on to the sliver of hope that some day you'll wake up to find it's all been a bad dream. Imagine you're driving down the same familiar street you drove down a hundred times before, past the hospital where a doctor removed your uterus. Except this time standing there at the intersection are women and men holding signs, protesting against the very thing that has altered your life.

That's exactly how many of the women driving by us feel. That's why they slow down, put on the breaks, roll down the windows. Many of the women who stumbled onto our protests told us they suddenly felt like they were caught up in a lie. And they were. An epic lie. The world's greatest secret. Some women feel exposed when they learn that some people are aware of the thing they've kept a secret, but at least now they acknowledge that the problems they're experiencing aren't going away, and they can begin to come to terms with it.

The most vulnerable time for hysterectomized women is two to six months after the surgery. For those who become suicidal, that's when they typically have their first thoughts of ending their lives. This suicidal ideation, as it's called, is a common response when women realize this is who they'll be for the rest of their lives. Maternal feelings and sexual feelings are diminished or gone. Women begin to feel like a burden to their family and friends. Doctors tell them there's nothing wrong with them, but they know they're not well.

More than 50% of the women HERS counsels say they've considered suicide. I get calls from people telling me their wife or mother or friend killed herself, because she didn't want to live with the aftermath. Their family or friends call HERS to find out if the suicide had something to do with the surgery. As hard as it is, they're grateful to finally know the truth of what led to her decision to forgo life with that pain, and to know it wasn't their fault. The blame falls squarely on the doctors who perform these barbaric surgeries and everyone who enables them.

One woman I counseled was in constant, debilitating pain after the surgery. She went to the doctor for stronger relief, but he refused to give her painkillers, accusing her of exaggerating her pain. Her husband wouldn't leave the house because he was afraid of what he'd find when he got home. Finally he had to go into work. After he left she thoroughly cleaned the house one last time and shot herself. He was sobbing when he called to tell me what happened. Although he didn't know how he could go on without her, he knew that she couldn't possibly go on that way.

The most common form of suicide is overdosing on pills. One woman I counseled threw herself in front of a bus. Many of the women I've counseled who I expected to see at the protests couldn't be reached. I called one woman I was sure would be at one of the protests, and her husband answered. "Nora," he said, "she killed herself when she lost her lawsuit. She felt it was just another abuse, and she just couldn't take it."

After Dolly Parton was hysterectomized, she was interviewed by Johann Hari. She told Hari, "Every day I thought, 'I wish I had the nerve to kill myself.'" Hari said, "At the same time, [Dolly's] weight ballooned," but that was obviously the least of her problems.[163]

Then the anger sets in. Anger is the beginning of the decision to live with it, to accept it, in one form or another. Either women choose to lie to themselves about it, which will gnaw at them in a different way, or they realize there's no point in continu-

---

[163] Hari, Johann, "It costs me a lot of money to look this cheap," *Evening Standard*, May 12, 2007.

ing the futile search for a remedy. They have the absolute knowledge that this is it. It may get worse, but it's not going to get better. The anger is what stops a lot of women from taking their lives. I begin to worry less about a woman I'm counseling when she shifts from grieving to angry. Then there's a good possibility she'll find a way to live with it.

Doctors tell women they have to let their anger go. In *un becoming*, the character Susan Herse realizes that Dr. Ridge hysterectomized and castrated her during exploratory surgery. Dr. Parker says, "Susan, it's very important that you don't overreact." Doctors don't acknowledge the aftermath they cause. If they did, it would be an admission that they know hysterectomy harms women.

The happy hysterectomy is all part of the greatest lie ever told. I tell women that anger is an important part of the process—the slow, dawning awareness. Contrary to Dr. Parker's advice in *un becoming*, I tell women to hold on to that anger. I'd worry about them more if they weren't angry. Their anger is justified and appropriate.

Each woman's circumstances are unique, but my message to anyone who talks about suicide is the same: "Don't let them silence you. Turn that anger toward helping other women. The damage can't be undone. But you can make a powerful difference in the lives of every intact woman by telling the truth about what the surgery has done to you."

A retired police officer from Las Vegas sent me an email describing herself as the "victim of a cut and slice ob/gyn who butchered me without cause." When women hit bottom and begin to search for a way to fight their way back up, invariably they ask me, "What can I do?"

My response is, "The reason to get up every day is your life is important. It matters. You have the power to make a change…to make a difference."

"But what can I do?" they ask me.

"It's up to every one of us. You can choose to do everything in your power to stop this from being done to other women. Soon we'll embark on a bold strategy to end this once and for all. When we do," I tell them, "we'll need everyone's support. We'll count on you to support changing the law. If you're not part of the solution you're part of the problem. It's up to you."

Sometimes women respond immediately with, "Of course I'll help!" For others, there's a pause. Through the phone line, this pause speaks volumes. I know they need a moment to dig deep down inside themselves, to fight back the tears and access that growing anger within them. When they do finally speak, it's from the heart. Invariably, they quietly, calmly and confidently say, "Yes. You can count on me."

FORTY-SIX

"un becoming addresses issues every woman should consider

before going under the knife."

Raleigh, North Carolina—Rick Schweikert

We spread out to cover the four corners of a busy intersection, but we needed three protestors on one of the corners to hand pamphlets out to the cars that lined up at the light. We propped up extra signs against the light poles down the block, so drivers would know why we were out there and could veer over to the curb to talk with us if they wanted to. One guy pulled his pickup over, yelling, "Here!" I circled the car, and he said angrily, "I need one of those," stressing the "I." When he took the pamphlet he kindly thanked me, but then the woman in the passenger seat snatched it from him as they raced away.

Raleigh was one of those places where if one of the cars up front took a pamphlet, everyone behind it would too. And if the first car didn't take one, sometimes no one behind them would.

As I ran down one of the long lines of cars with hands waving out their windows impatiently waiting for a pamphlet, the driver of an SUV said, "Can't you see I've got children in here?" I wasn't sure if that meant she wanted me to go away or if she wanted me to hurry up, but then she flipped me off. There were four or five children in her car. I wanted to ask her why it wasn't okay to say the H word in front of her children, but it was somehow okay to give the bird to a complete stranger. Instead I just moved on to the next car, but before I could the driver of the SUV cranked her steering wheel over and gunned her engine like she was trying to run me over. I jumped out of the way, which would've put me in the way of an oncoming car, except that the other driver saw the whole thing and paused. When I got back to the curb safely, the people in the car looking out for me put their window down. I handed the woman in the passenger seat a pamphlet as the driver leaned over her, saying, "That was a close one!" And then the woman in the passenger seat gave me the usual, "God bless you," as they drove away.

And that for me was pretty much the Raleigh protest in a nutshell: One person wanted to run me down for subjecting her children to a medical term, and another person god-blessed me for dodging traffic to get information out to the public.

In addition to an unexpected cold snap, that night a steady drizzle fell on the Smoky Mountains, which made for some slippery roads in the morning. I wasn't sure we'd make it driving to the protest, but we did. There was a lot less traffic than the day before, but because it was Sunday in the Bible Belt we still managed to distribute a few more boxes of information.

A mini-van veered over quickly to the curb. I jumped back because I was still a little gun shy from the woman who tried to run me down the day before. The driver put her window down, asking, "What's this all about?" I told her, and she said, "Well I'm scheduled for one the day after tomorrow!"

I called Nora over. As Nora spoke with her, the cars behind her honked their horns for her to push off, but she was intent on hearing what Nora had to say. Beside a busy highway, on a frigid, icy January morning, Nora was able to provide the woman with information she needed to make an informed decision—the information a doctor she was paying her hard earned money to wouldn't.

Something's wrong with this picture, I thought—free accurate information versus costly lies. She asked a few more questions and then confirmed the HERS contact information on the pamphlet so she could get in touch with Nora after she made a call to the gynecologist. "Because I'm damned well going to cancel my surgery!" she said.

Negotiators sometimes say if you're not *at* the table you're *on* the table. That certainly holds true for hysterectomy. If you're not active in the discussion, and if you don't know your options going in, you're in an extremely vulnerable position. Another thing negotiators say is to not come to the table if you don't like the menu. If hysterectomy is the only option, then you'd better find a different doctor.

The reading of *un becoming* in North Carolina took place after the Sunday protest at Meredith College, directed by Steven Roten on behalf of Stillwater Theatre, which produced a fine performance. Afterwards a local radio program interviewed us, and we received a handful of emails from people who saw a review of the reading in "Robert's Reviews."

> … The Still Water Theatre production of Schweikert's provocative play, sponsored by the HERS Foundation and presented as a free staged reading last Sunday afternoon at Meredith College in Raleigh, NC, deserved a much larger audience and more local news media coverage than it received. The cast assembled—and superbly orchestrated—by director Steven Roten included some of the Triangle's finest actors… If you are a woman—or anyone who has a mother or wife or sister or daughter or female relative or friend—Un Becoming is a vitally important play to bring to her attention. Certainly, it addresses issues that every woman should consider before going under the knife. The price of uninformed consent can be, quite literally, unbearable.[164]

[164] McDowell, Robert, "Un Becoming Exposes the Damage Done by Unnecessary Hysterectomies," *Robert's Reviews*, January 30, 2005.

FORTY-SEVEN

"The map is not the territory."

Phoenix, Arizona—Nora W. Coffey

In 2004, 11,105 women were reported to have been hysterectomized in the Grand Canyon State, and 8,790 were castrated.[165] The Patient Education Institute's X-Plain hysterectomy tutorial on the National Library of Medicine website calls hysterectomy "very safe."[166] While it may be true that most women survive the surgery, leaving the operating room breathing doesn't make hysterectomy safe.

The Arizona protest took place at St. Joseph's Hospital and Medical Center, one of 42 hospitals comprising Catholic Healthcare West, the eighth largest hospital chain in America, and growing.[167] The "expansion" project of St. Joseph's was bigger than the main building.

Like Albuquerque, the residents of Phoenix seemed nervous about someone approaching their car. If their window was down, many of them quickly put it up, something we didn't encounter very much elsewhere. Later, I felt the need to get out of the city. To be somewhere with no hospitals…a place where there was no such thing as hysterectomy.

Once I got outside the city, I found myself driving along what is referred to as a "minimum maintenance road." It was

---

[165] "Number of All-Listed Procedures by Category and Age Group, Arizona, 2004," *Arizona Department of Health Services*, http://azdhs.gov/plan/hip/by/procedure/2004/proc104.xls, July 12, 2007.
[166] "Hysterectomy," tutorial, *X-Plain.com*, Patient Education Institute.
[167] "Success Story: Catholic Healthcare West," *Novell*, http://www.novell.com/collateral/4681012/4681012.pdf.

unpaved in parts, and soon I was driving only on gravel, and then clay, and more than once I approached a sudden sharp turn in the road that was unmarked.

Around one of the bends in that treacherous road I came upon Bumble Bee, Arizona, comprised of about half a dozen trailer homes and two buildings—the Bumble Bee School and the Bumble Bee Bar. Having found the isolation I was looking for, I was now glad to find some sign of life.

Every resident of Bumble Bee must've been huddled in that tiny bar. They stared as if a ghost had just walked through the door, until a man named Virgil ceremoniously vacated his bar stool for me. His merry blue eyes flashed when he welcomed me to "little old Bumble Bee," as he called it.

There was a wooden column at one corner of the bar with business cards, comics, and quotations pinned to it. One of the business cards advertised the services of a plumber and was printed in fluorescent pink, with a quote from the British columnist Julie Burchill: "Four things a woman should know: How to look like a girl, how to act like a lady, how to think like a man, and how to work like a dog." Aside from being fluorescent pink, it caught my eye because Rick also borrowed this line for the song he wrote for *un becoming*: "To get ahead these days / a woman's gotta look like a girl, / she's got to act like a man, / work like a dog, / and find the joy in the Joy of Cooking."

I felt like I'd been dropped onto the set of a Sam Shepard play. The women were guarded, even angry at the attention I was getting from the men. One of them boisterously talked about her physically abusive husband. The bartender never smiled, eyeing me suspiciously. I asked him if I could take the plumber's business card to show Rick, and he caught me off guard when he flatly said, "No."

"What's a woman doing alone out here in the mountains?" Virgil asked.

"Are the mountains any less risky for men?" I asked.

He laughed, introduced me to everyone in the bar, and then I told them about the protest. Virgil seemed interested in learning more, and not at all embarrassed by the information.

The women at the tables began to let their guard down. One of them said, referring to the protest, "It's good there're people out there who care enough about women to do that."

After I finished my drink, just as ceremoniously as Virgil had offered his barstool to me, I offered it back to him. I shook their hands goodbye, and I left.

From there I drove to Crown King. Only slightly larger than Bumble Bee, it did have a restaurant. I sat near two young couples with children. The men kept to themselves as one of the women spoke softly to the other about all the medical problems she was having since her last baby was born. She kept an eye on the men, making sure not to talk too loudly, using awkward euphemisms about her female organs.

It was enough to watch their feet to get a sense of what was going on. She and her husband fidgeted nervously, while the feet of the other couple remained firmly planted on the floor. The woman who was speaking wore black pumps with little black bows. Her pumps shifted exactly at the same moment that her husband's work boots did. He was trying to hear what she was saying to her friend, but he didn't want her to know he was listening-in. He made sure to never look at them, but he leaned their way to catch what they were saying and wasn't at all attentive to his buddy across the table. Because of where I was sitting, I couldn't help but catch a word or two. That, combined with the secrecy and body language clues, made it obvious that the woman in the black pumps had been hysterectomized.

This can't be, I thought. I made a conscious decision to escape it all for one evening, but nowhere, not even in remote Crown King, Arizona, are women safe from gynecology. Clearly, she needed someone to talk with about what she was going through, and her husband needed to talk with someone about their relationship since the surgery. But she whispered to make sure he didn't hear her, and he eavesdropped rather than just coming right out and talking with her.

Many partners of hysterectomized women have told me something like, "She says everything's okay one day, and then she's angry and won't speak to me the next. What I do on Monday seems okay, but it isn't okay on Tuesday. One day she tells me she appreciates how much I care, and then I say the same thing the next day and she says I don't understand."

The best advice I can give them is to back off. "I understand" are the two most helpful words you can to a hysterectomized woman. And letting a woman know you're angry about what was done to her without her consent is important too—that you understand that the hysterectomy may not be the end of her medical problems, only the beginning…that her ailments aren't character flaws but symptoms of the biological havoc wrought by the surgery.

Efforts made to cheer up a hysterectomized woman the way that you once did may not work anymore, because she's different. She may not find the same things funny. Family outings, holidays, even a vacation trip may no longer be fun—they may be too physically exhausting and emotionally draining. She may weep at a gift that once brought joy.

A while later I was in the restroom, and I recognized the woman's black pumps with the bows under the stall beside me. "Excuse me," I said. "I'm sorry, because it wasn't my intention to overhear your conversation, but this is what I do." I took a pamphlet from my bag and handed it to her under the stall. "If you need information, this might help."

She took the pamphlet and was silent a moment, before saying, "Look, I'm okay, all right?" I took my time in case she wanted to ask me something, but she didn't say anything else.

As I asked for my bill and prepared to leave, the comments from the other woman at the table seemed to indicate that she was a nurse. She was no help, because she seemed to accept everything the doctors told her friend as gospel. This was something I saw a lot of, especially in rural areas. Because everyone knows each other in a small community, and because most of them are relatives or friends, nurses are more apt to support whatever the doctor advises, and much less likely to disagree. Rural people seem to go to doctors less than people in the city, but when they do some of them are more likely to do what they're told and to accept it without question. In many of rural towns, doctors come to visit once every 30 to 60 days. A woman experiencing heavy menstrual bleeding, uterine prolapse, or pelvic pain knows that if she doesn't take the doctor's recommendation she'll have to live with her symptoms for another month or two. This creates a false sense of urgency—a need to do something now, while the doctor's in town.

"Tonight was essential," I wrote Rick in an email. "It renewed me. Although a mountain lion made me rethink sleeping under the stars and I had to travel treacherous, moonless roads back to a stuffy hotel room, tonight I'm more determined than ever to stop what's being done to women."

FORTY-EIGHT

Joan Rivers: "Liars: hysterectomy didn't improve sex life."

Dallas, Texas—Rick Schweikert

Total number of hysterectomies in the state of Texas:

Year	Hysterectomies
1999	40,537
2000	44,249
2001	47,358

Regional hysterectomy rate variation, per 100 women aged 18-64:

State of Texas:	10.01
East Texas, Texas:	8.31
Waco, Texas:	12.96
Dallas, Texas:	10.52[168]

According to these statistics, the hysterectomy rate throughout the state of Texas increased about 17% in the three years between 1999 and 2001. And that data doesn't include outpatient hysterectomies, which is discussed in the final chapter. Just as there are regional variations around the country, the hysterectomy rate in Waco is about 56% higher than it is in East Texas, about a three-hour drive away.

Joan, Debbie, and a few others joined us at the Presbyterian Hospital in suburban Dallas. Here's a diary entry from the inestimable Joan:

> In mid-February I traveled to Texas for the protest at the Presbyterian Hospital of Dallas. I had

---

[168] "Utilization of Specific Inpatient Procedures by Texas Hospital Referral Region, 1999-2001," Texas Hospital Inpatient Discharge Data, Texas Health Care Information Council.

great difficulty finding a hotel room because of the 30,000+ person HIMMS (Healthcare Information Medical Management Systems) convention. The first morning I stepped into the hotel elevator and a gentleman asked me if I was with the HIMMS group. "No I'm not with the HIMMS group," I replied, "I'm with the HERS group." He laughed, so I asked him if he knew what HERS was. He said he thought I was joking. I said "No, it's the Hysterectomy Educational Resources & Services Foundation," and gave him the HERS brochures.

Nora and I stationed ourselves on a corner by a bus stop opposite the front entrance of the Presbyterian Hospital. Although the pedestrian traffic was light, there was plenty of automobile traffic. We distributed the literature when the cars stopped for the light, and most drivers were grateful. Some bus drivers even accepted stacks of brochures for their passengers. We also encountered a few women on the street who told us of their personal stories of how damaged they were by a hysterectomy. I found out that the hospital had a Lymphedema Clinic and I stopped in to visit a Manual Lymph Drainage therapist. I informed her of the HERS protest. She was happy to accept the educational brochures.

Nora invited me to lunch with a newspaper reporter who had requested an interview with her which lasted two hours. I found it very interesting. Her husband is a well-known Dallas radio talk show host. Nora gives a really good interview.

An undercover police officer showed up, asked for a pamphlet, read it while sitting there in her car, thanked us, and said she'd try to attend the reading of the play that night at the Grace United Methodist Church.

Having produced readings of *Vagina Monologues*, Melodie Minshew and Barbara Miller offered to organize the *un becoming* reading in Dallas. We now knew we'd get through the year as planned with only one more reading in Atlanta before the full production in Washington, DC.

During the talkback, Melodie said, "Everything you say makes sense, but I still don't understand why no one's talking about this."

"A whole lot of doctors have spoken and written about hysterectomy abuse," I said, "going back hundreds of years. Most of the books and articles I've read about how hospitals are dangerous places were written by doctors. It's a long, sad history, but maybe what you're asking is, 'If hysterectomy is so common, can it really be all that bad?'"

It's a valid question that leads to more questions. For example, can lobotomy really be all that bad for you if Antonio Egas Moniz, one of its pioneers, won the Nobel prize for "perfecting" it, and he and others went on to make it a common procedure, literally scrambling the brains of more than 50,000 American women and children? Lobotomy was praised as a miracle cure by the doctors who performed it, and it was condemned as a barbaric, harmful, and unscientific experimentation by those who fought to stop it.[169] Mary Daly gives an example of someone who was said to have been improved by psychosurgery:

> They report that psychosurgery performed on a woman patient was successful, despite the fact that she killed herself. Her suicide was interpreted as a sign that she was getting

[169] Gajilan, Chris, "Survivor recounts lobotomy at age 12, Procedure once considered legitimate medical treatment, *CNN*, November 30, 2005; Weiner Eric, "Nobel Panel Urged to Rescind Prize for Lobotomies," *NPR, Day to Day*, August 10, 2005.

over her depression, a "gratifying" effect of the operation.[170]

Moniz's career was cut short when one of his own "success stories" shot him in the back, paralyzing him for life. I saw the 1982 movie "Frances" about the actress Frances Farmer. But "Frances" was filmed five years after Congress formed the National Committee for the Protection of Human Subjects of Biomedical and Behavioral Research to investigate psychosurgery, and several states had already illegalized lobotomy…27 years after it was banned in Russia.

"And what about DES?" I asked the audience, referring to diethylstilbestrol, the drug that doctors routinely prescribed to pregnant women from 1938 to 1971 to prevent miscarriages. "After all, more than ten million women were exposed to it by their doctors." In her foreword to *DES Stories*, Margaret Lee Braun writes:

> DES is linked to cancer and reproductive injuries in the daughters and sons exposed *in utero,* and in the mothers prescribed the drug. DES daughters have higher rates of vaginal and cervical cancer; increased incidence of reproductive problems, such as infertility, ectopic pregnancies, miscarriage, and premature delivery; and possible autoimmune problems. DES sons have a higher incidence of reproductive anomalies, including underdeveloped and undescended testicles, epididymal cysts, and structural changes. DES mothers have a higher incidence of breast cancer.[171]
> DES was banned for use in pregnancies in 1971.

Someone else in the audience asked why there was no media coverage in Dallas for the Protest & Play. "It did make it onto

[170]   Daly, Mary, *GYN/ECOLOGY*, Beacon, 1990.
[171]   Braun, Margaret Lee, *DES Stories*, Visual Studies Workshop, 2001.

some of the calendar listings," Nora said, "but it's true that we haven't gotten any media coverage in Dallas other than that."

Nora mentioned the newspaper interview Joan refers to in her journal entry above, but the article was never published. And as Joan said, the newspaper reporter's husband was Glenn Mitchell—one of Dallas' best-known radio personalities. Nora was also interviewed by Glenn, but the interview didn't air until after the protest.

Glenn's show was hosted by KERA 90.1, the National Public Radio affiliate for Dallas. About a week before the interview, Nora got a call from the show's producer. As she does before every interview, Nora asked him who else would be on the program. He said there'd be no one else on the show with Nora except Glenn. He then went on to say the interview would be brief and would dovetail with a whole week of programming they were doing on the topic of health and fitness.

Immediately Nora's antenna went up. Whenever medicine is the topic—whether it's free wellness checkups, a study about female sexuality after hysterectomy, or a media interview with a doctor—you can almost always follow the money to a big corporation funding it for reasons related to profit, not health. Quite often, Nora told the audience at the Dallas reading, it's as subtle as a pleasant voice telling us, "This program was brought to you by Johnson & Johnson"—or Pfizer, or GlaxoSmithKline, or Biosphere.

"So," Nora said to the producer, "a health fair on a public radio station? Why don't you tell me a little bit about it. Who's sponsoring it?"

The producer said a local hospital was involved, but he hesitated, saying, "Well you know, it's not exactly sponsored by them, but they're participating."

"In what way are they participating?" Nora asked. "Is this a health fair that was the idea of the producers at KERA, or is this paid advertisement?"

"No, we've been doing these things for years, and public radio doesn't do paid advertisement. Presbyterian is just one of the lead participants."

"That's very interesting," Nora said, "because the reason we'll be in Dallas is we'll be holding a protest against unconsented hysterectomy at Presbyterian Hospital."

He fell silent. After a long pause, he said, "I need to call you right back."

While she waited, Nora got onto the Presbyterian website and found the following, which was also reported in the *Dallas Morning News*:

Healthy Women, Healthy Lives

Date:	2/12/2005 8:30 a.m. to 3:00 p.m.
Location:	Adams Mark Hotel, Dallas
Description:	Join Presbyterian Healthcare System and KERA for Healthy Women, Healthy Lives at the Adams Mark Hotel in Dallas, Texas on Saturday, February 12, 2005 from 8:30 a.m. to 3:00 p.m.
	Cost is $35 per person and includes continental breakfast, luncheon, keynote speaker, three breakout sessions, health screenings and a gift bag.

For reservations, please call 1-800-4-Presby.

About five minutes later, the producer called back. He said, "Nora, we're going to have to interview you another day. The medical center is sponsoring our health fair, and it would really look like we were trying to set the hospital up."

"But I thought they weren't sponsoring it."

"No, they are sponsoring it," he said, "but I'm sure Glenn would like to have you on his show some other day."

KERA's website says they've been hosting these corporate-sponsored events for years:

> Since 1999, nearly 7,000 North Texans have attended the KERA-sponsored health seminars, which offer attendees the opportunity to hear from - and question - experts with advice about how to feel better, stay healthier and be more informed about health issues.

Some of the sponsors have included AstraZeneca Pharmaceuticals, GlaxoSmithKline, and Harris Methodist Hospital. Harris is part of the Texas Health Resources, Inc. (THR) chain of hospitals, which includes Presbyterian, the site of our protest. THR's website, Texashealth.org, says it's "one o of the largest faith-based, nonprofit health care delivery systems in the United States."

> ✓   The system serves more than 6.3 million people living in 29 counties in north central Texas... THR was formed in 1997 with the merger of Fort Worth-based Harris Methodist Health System and Dallas-based Presbyterian Healthcare Resources. Later that year, Arlington Memorial Hospital joined the THR system... More than 18,250 employees... More than 3,600 physicians with staff privileges... 27 health care sites... More than 2,600 licensed hospital beds... $5B in sales.

So Nora called Glenn. "NPR says it's a public broadcasting company that doesn't take money for paid advertisements and that your reporting is unbiased and balanced," Nora said. "But your health fair is paid for by the hospital, so it's advertising by any other name, is it not?"

Glenn didn't deny it, saying only, "If we interview you at the time we had scheduled, it could cost us our jobs, Nora. Can we get you on the show in a couple of weeks?"

While we were protesting the next day, Nora counseled a woman from Dallas. I'll call her Margaret. During the counseling session, Margaret sobbed and screamed for fifteen minutes before her husband took the phone. He too was beside himself, because there was nothing he could do to help his wife. Nora said their disbelief that the aftermath was permanent was heartbreaking, made worse by the fact that several of their friends who'd had the surgery encouraged Margaret to have it. Each one said they were just fine after the surgery. Margaret might have asked herself, can hysterectomy really be all that bad if all these women underwent it and no one's telling her not to go through with it?

So after the surgery, Margaret and her husband called their friends back to tell them about all the problems Margaret was having. Did they have any clues why Margaret was in such bad shape, they asked their friends? Each one in her own way said they too were suffering the same problems since the surgery as Margaret, but they didn't want to mention it. Margaret and her husband asked, "How could our own friends do this to us?"

There are many women whose accomplishments after the surgery are impressive, such as Liz Taylor, U.S. Senator Dianne Feinstein, comedienne Joan Rivers (who's own entry in *Six Word Memoirs* is, "Liars: hysterectomy didn't improve sex life."[172]), and homemaking advocate and business magnate Martha Stewart. It's a testimony to what some women can endure.

---

[172] Smith, Larry, *Six Word Memoirs*, HarperCollins, 2008.

FORTY-NINE

"The conversion of normal, healthy people into patients."

Honolulu, Hawaii—Nora W. Coffey

"Nora," the office assistant informs me, "your nine o'clock appointment is on hold." I pick up the phone as I have many, many thousands of times before, and say, "This is Nora Coffey, how may I help you?"

The caller introduces herself to me in her most formal tone, telling me that she "had to have" the surgery and is only interested in getting some information about how to deal with some problems she's having. She's suspicious of me, but she slowly opens up as I reassure her that our conversation is confidential. "It's just that it's not easy finding anyone who understands," she says, "you know?" And with that she's suddenly vulnerable and unsure of herself. I've now been on the phone with this complete stranger for less than a minute, but her guard is fading and giving way to tears.

When she gathers herself, I ask her to start at the beginning. She explains how one day she was fine, and the next day after a Pap smear her doctor said something about a hysterectomy. Then she begins to lose focus and her thoughts become scattered, partly because she's embarrassed to realize that she's not familiar enough with her own anatomy to tell me exactly what was done to her.

Her friends and family don't understand why she doesn't just "get over it." Her doctor claims he doesn't understand why she's having so many problems either, saying, "None of my other patients have any of these problems." But she suspects he's lying.

A slow realization has begun to dawn on her—what the doctor told her before the surgery means nothing. It's what the doctor didn't tell her that suddenly means everything. The doctor told her the hysterectomy would be routine. "It didn't even occur to me to get a second opinion," she says. "I figured it would be great, no more periods." Now her wariness turns to anger as she says, "My periods weren't that big of a deal."

From the very first moment she broke through the fog of anesthesia, she realized everything was different. "When I got home no one looked at me the same way," she says. "But then I realized—they're not the ones who've changed…it's me. I need you to help me get back to my old self again." She says she'll send HERS her medical records and make another appointment. She apologizes for crying, and tells me next time she'll be better. I tell her she never has to apologize to me.

Another caller has fibroids. She was told hysterectomy was her only choice, because they were too big to remove without taking out her uterus. A gynecologist said she doesn't need her uterus or ovaries because she's 42 years old and isn't planning on having more children. I refer her to a gynecologist who has consistently good outcomes performing myomectomies. She's one caller who won't become another hysterectomy statistic.

"For me, the joys of life have been replaced with pain and suffering," the next caller tells me. And then between calls I open a letter that says, "Please help me, I really think I'm starting to lose it." And then an email drops into my inbox—"I avoid friends and public places since my surgery. Please tell me how to deal with this." And then my ten o'clock appointment marvels at her own words when she realizes, "Before the surgery, the door to my home was always open, entertaining friends and family late into the night. But now my door's always locked...curtains drawn."

One caller hurries to tell me everything about herself before her appointment is over, as the next caller patiently holds the line, waiting to tell me how it was done to her. And another, and another. There are a lot of gynecologists out there, but there's just one HERS Foundation.

Of the women who contact HERS who were told they need a hysterectomy or who've already been hysterectomized, the fastest growing age group is 17-25. The youngest woman I've spoken with was 11 at the time of the surgery. The worst part about her story wasn't that her mother asked a doctor to hysterectomize and sterilize her daughter. The worst part about it was that the doctor and nurses went ahead and performed the surgery on an innocent child, amputating her reproductive sex organs without any indication of disease or medical problems. They did it because her mother was afraid that her daughter, one of her 12 children, would repeat the same "mistakes" she had made in life. It wasn't until decades later that the girl, now an adult woman but stunted by the effects of hysterectomy, finally found HERS and realized what was done to her. She vividly recalled every moment leading up to the surgery.

I dream of a country where all hospitals—whether they're affiliated with Johns Hopkins or the University of Hawaii—are shut down for harming any woman or any man of any age.

Long before HERS' 48th protest was planned in the 50th state, I knew that women on the edenic Hawaiian Islands weren't any safer from doctors than women anywhere else. Maybe less so, because Polynesian women are geographically isolated and many can't afford to travel beyond their own island.

Many Hawaiian women have contacted HERS throughout the years. From my perspective, a call to HERS from Pukalani might as well come from Poughkeepsie. What differentiates a call from a woman in one part of the world from another doesn't become apparent until you visit those places first hand.

I can refer a woman in Baltimore to a doctor in Philadelphia, knowing she probably won't have too much trouble getting there. I also know a doctor in Hawaii who I feel comfortable referring women to, but his practice is on the "big island" of Oahu. It wasn't until I visited Hawaii that I understood that many Hawaiians never leave the island of their birth.

Rick and I recently spoke at the National Women's Studies Association conference in Chicago. In the Q&A that followed, a young woman from Hawaii told us that her doctor dropped her as "his patient" because she questioned his recommendation for hysterectomy. It's a common story. When she sought a new gynecologist to examine her, she couldn't get an appointment. And every other doctor on the island followed suit. "Do you think I was blacklisted for being an uncooperative patient?" she asked. She had the means to fly to the mainland to find a doctor who'd treat her conservatively, but most of the women I've counseled in Hawaii aren't able to do that.

The Kingdom of Hawaii was unified by King Kamehameha the Great in 1810. Esther Kapiolani was the granddaughter of the last king of Kauai and reigned as Queen Consort until the islands were annexed by the United States in 1898. The Kapiolani Medical Center For Women & Children was named for her.[173] Women's hospitals and women's clinics are proliferating, but Polynesian

---

[173] http://www.kapiolani.org/women-and-children/about-us/default.aspx.

women don't need medical centers and clinics to poke, probe, and explore their bodies any more than Polynesian men do.

The fact is, gynecology is a dangerous specialty. Both men and women age, and in the aging process they both experience urogenital changes. Some of them lead to the common inconveniences of any aging body, but they rarely become medical problems until a doctor makes them so. There are menopause clinics for women, but imagine your father seeking counseling for urinary problems, testosterone deficiency, and sagging breasts as he aged. These are conditions commonly seen in aging men, but there are no men's hospitals named after Hawaiian kings that focus on male organs.

As they are elsewhere, women are the biggest consumers of the Hawaiian health industry. Doctors, hospitals, device manufacturers, and pharmaceutical companies market themselves more to women than men—from plastic surgery to hormones to adult diapers. Early feminists had good intentions when they fought for equal healthcare for women, but that's been turned on its head by gynecology. The growing "women's health" industry is working against women.

A good example of how and why women are targeted is evident in gynecology's latest and most celebrated medical money-maker—uterine artery (or fibroid) embolization, otherwise known as UAE or UFE, which is addressed in our Colorado chapter. In a *Journal of Vascular Interventional Radiology* article, whose lead author is an 'MD, MBA,' the authors describe their success marketing this surgery to their patients.

> The authors tested the hypothesis that an advertising strategy focused on a defined target market can expand an existing uterine fibroid embolization practice... Based on the analysis

the authors determined that the target audience
was professional black women aged 35 to 45...
The 17 extra cases performed over 3 months
represented a 27% increase in case volume...
This resulted in a net revenue gain $50,317 and
a nonannualized rate of return of approximately
625%... As Interventional Radiologists look to
develop and expand existing practices, tradi-
tional marketing tools such as those utilized
in this study can be used to facilitate practice
growth for specific clinical programs, such as
uterine artery embolization. Defining a target
market can significantly expand an existing
uterine fibroid embolization practice... The
study was assisted by the aid of a single industrial
partner, Biosphere, who provided financial and
strategic resources... Our marketing analysis of
the current uterine fibroid market strongly suggests that a direct advertising approach would
be successful... The net profit can be divided by
certain variables to obtain certain benchmarks
such as average profit per call ($559), average
profit per clinic visit ($1438), average profit per
case performed ($2959) and average profit per
week of advertising ($6289).[174]

Simply by pushing UAE, doctors can pump an *additional*
$6,289 per week (or $327,028 a year) into their practice. This
may be good news for profit-minded doctors, but it's bad news
for women. This study is a clear case of conflict of interest, due to
the fact that Biosphere Medical, a company that manufactures tiny
plastic balls that are injected into women's uterine arteries during UAE, helped pay for it. This article clearly demonstrates the

[174] Howard B. Chrisman, et. al., "The Positive Effect of Targeted Marketing on an
Existing Uterine Fibroid Embolization Practice," *Journal of Vascular Interventional
Radiology*, March 2006.

extent to which the health and wellbeing of women are secondary to profit.

Like most hospitals today, the advertising I saw for the Kapiolani Hospital did little to promote itself as a place women go to for medical problems. Its advertisements were similar to those of the nearby resorts and hotels. Their website offers expectant couples a "FREE Having A Baby Kit and $30.00 Gift Certificate."[175] Until Obstetrics and Gynecology wedged its way into our lives, women never needed having-a-baby kits. Another example of medical marketing is the hospital's 'Kapiolani Babies On-Line,' "a free birth announcement that provides parents a safe and easy way to announce their new little addition via the Internet."[176] But since when was announcing the birth of a baby difficult or unsafe? And what does this service have to do with healing? Nothing. But it has everything to do with profits.

Homebirth advocate Dr. Mayer Eisenstein put it this way:

> Could the hospital be changed and somehow become as safe as home for laboring women? The answer is 'No.' There is something about just walking into a hospital that changes the dynamics of labor. The length of labor is significantly increased in the hospital... The safety of home birth, which is something I have always believed on an intuitive level, is explainable through statistical data [but also because women who homebirth] have the home court advantage."[177]

---

[175] https://www.kapiolani.org/women-and-children/health-services-for-women/having-a-baby-kit.aspx.
[176] http://www.kapiolani.org/women-and-children/health-services-for-women/maternity-and-newborn-care/kapiolani-babies-on-line.aspx.
[177] Eisenstein, Mayer, *Homefirst Health Services*, http://www.homefirst.com/faqs/examples/homebirth.html.

A major shift in medicine has occurred in this country right under our noses. In <u>The Social Transformation of American Medicine</u>, Paul Starr writes:

> The failure to rationalize medical services under public control meant that sooner or later they would be rationalized under private control. Instead of public regulation, there will be private regulation, and instead of public planning, there will be corporate planning.

Whereas the sick were once treated by a healing profession, that profession now operates under the corporate web of intense competition. It has become a selling profession, and sales are good. Hawaiian women, for example, might want to shop around, because the competing women's hospital next door might give them a $40 gift certificate and sheets with a better thread count with even safer and easier baby announcements than Kapiolani.

Kapiolani seems to focus on maternal services, but they advertise 197 hospital beds compared to only 90 bassinets.[178] An October 2007 report in *Crain's Chicago Business* about a new women's hospital is telling:

> The Oct. 20 opening of Northwestern Memorial Healthcare's gleaming new women's hospital will cement its identity as Chicago's maternity mecca—but delivering babies won't deliver profits. Instead, executives expect the influx of moms and babies…to feed an expanded menu of more-profitable medical services…in 10 sleek operating rooms where doctors will perform gynecological and breast surgeries, among the most lucrative procedures in women's medicine… Maternity wards have long been loss

---

[178]   http://www.punahou.edu/uploaded/pdf/alumni/KapiolaniHealthBoard.pdf.

leaders for hospitals... Mr. Harrison and Northwestern are betting they can turn a profit on deliveries indirectly by locking in moms and their
new families as lifelong hospital customers. [179]

Hospitals make a profit convincing you that doctors, not
women, deliver babies, and then they make the real money from
procedures and treatments they sell women along the assembly
line of women's health, for the rest of their lives.

As Eugene D. Robin says in *Matters of Life & Death: Risks vs.
Benefits of Medical Care,* "Many of the practices of modern medicine
result in the conversion of normal, healthy people into patients."
He goes on to say that most medical interventions appear to have
little positive impact on health:

> Many are untested and some are either harm-
> ful or have unacceptably high risks. Remember
> that life is to be lived. It is far too short to be
> lived in a state of obsession with the possibil-
> ity or the prevention of disease. Not only is an
> ounce of prevention not terribly effective; it can
> cause a pound or more of distraction. Perhaps
> Ben Franklin was right—'Nothing is more fatal
> to health than overcare of it.'[180]

The Kapiolani Women's Center website advertises "free"
osteoporosis information sessions, monthly menopause lectures,
weight loss programs (with cooking classes "led by physician"),
incontinence testing, ultrasounds, diabetes counseling, sports
nutrition counseling, counseling to help women cope with major
life changes, botox, hair removal, massage, heart health information sessions, endometriosis support groups, and so on. But if you

---

[179] Michael Colias, "Betting On Baby", *Crain's Chicago Business,* Oct. 8, 2007.
[180] Robin, Eugene D., *Matters of Life & Death: Risks vs. Benefits of Medical Care,*
W H Freeman & Company, 1984.

search Kapiolani's online "Health Guide" for information about "hysterectomy" you'll find the usual unreliable information, misinformation, and omissions of fact that you'll find on other hospital websites.

A study of newspaper ads placed by 17 'top-rated university medical centers' published in *Archives of Internal Medicine* highlights the conflict between motives of promoting public health and making money.

> Some ads, especially those touting specific services, might create a sense of need in otherwise healthy patients and "seem to put the financial interests of the academic medical center ahead of the best interests of the patients."[181]

It's no wonder that, as Ivan Illich says, "Unnecessary surgery is a standard procedure."[182]

My daughter Jessica met me in Hawaii, but she was exhausted from a demanding work schedule so I tried not to wake her when I headed out to get the Honolulu protest underway. I didn't expect anyone else to join me, because I got no responses from the women I've counseled on Oahu.

There were plenty of cars entering and leaving the hospital parking garage, but there were almost no pedestrians. So I packed everything back up and decided to investigate other ways of getting the word out.

I usually avoided parking on hospital private property, but I didn't see any police or security, so I followed the traffic inside Kapiolani's garage. Much like the ninth-floor entrance to the hos-

---

[181] Wade, Rick, "Study Raises Question About Hospital Advertising," *USA Today*, March 8, 2005.
[182] Illich, Ivan, *Medical Nemesis*, Pantheon, 1982.

pital in Portland, I spotted an entrance to the hospital inside the garage.

Most of the people who passed by seemed poor. And I never saw so many babies. A lot of the women were obese. It's difficult to separate cultural differences from economic and political factors, but you get a pretty good feeling about people when you do what I do for as long as I have. The women I met weren't stressed out, really, but there was more of a downtrodden feel to them…the other side of the sun-and-surf of tourism. These were the native Hawaiians, as opposed to the hordes of tourists who sent postcards of tropical paradise back to the mainland.

During one of the brief lulls in foot traffic, I began papering parked cars. A lot of the cars had objects hanging from their rearview mirrors—some Christian symbols, but mostly natural objects like feathers and a lot of woven symbols like what we saw in the Dakotas. No one spoke to me. I watched them slide the pamphlets out from under their windshield wipers. I didn't detect any change in expression as they read them.

When I was done for the day I took a look around inside the hospital. Kapiolani was dirty and deteriorated. As I drove my car out of the parking garage past the hospital back toward our hotel, I thought, "This is the depressing place our society has chosen to bring children into the world?"

That night we went to a restaurant that was highly recommended. A woman sat at the table across from us with a man decked out in full military dress uniform. Ribbons and medals and stripes dangled from his chest and shoulders. He asked what we were doing in Hawaii. It was interesting watching their expressions change when I told them that although we hoped to see the sights

I was there to conduct a protest against unconsented hysterectomy. The doctor was unfazed. Without hesitation he congratulated me, readily acknowledging that hysterectomy was a serious problem on the islands. "Particularly in the military," he said.

His wife told us about hysterectomized women she knew in Hawaii who were having a hard time. "Like everything else on the islands, even access to information can be a struggle," she said. "It's something that's just not talked about here."

In our hotel room I could feel that it was shocking and worrisome for Jessica to see the changes in my body since the last time we were together. Jessica's an industrial designer with an interest in universal design products. She couldn't help but notice the continued compression in my spine and the increased bow of my back from the surgery almost 25 years before. "I'm the incredible shrinking woman," I said. "There aren't any adult sizes smaller than zero."

Jessica understood the significance of this. Because there wasn't anything I could do about it, she simply took in the information without uttering a word. But I could sense the hurt and concern in her to see these changes in her mother's body, that each year take a greater toll on me.

I was having trouble with my hip, and it was nice how natural it was for her to accommodate me. When we walked, she slowed her pace to match mine. I realized then more than ever how special that is. Helping without asking—it's what we raise our children to do.

My children and I don't talk about the surgery, but I sometimes wonder if they remember who I was before the surgery. Following my "incredible shrinking woman" comment, it seemed like

Jessica wanted to talk more about it. And because I was there for a protest, not a vacation, and since our conversations were frequently interrupted by urgent counseling calls, I felt comfortable broaching the subject with her.

"Do you remember who I was before?" I asked her. "Not just as a mother, but as a woman living her life?"

She looked hurt by the question, and I immediately regretted asking it. But then she said, "Mom…? Of course I do!" And then she paused, before saying, "We used to dance to *Bad, Bad Leroy Brown* in the living room!"

Jessica remembered when my life was filled with artists and activists—our house was always bustling with the laughter of friends stopping by with a stranger in tow, staying for dinner, sometimes sleeping on couches, some of them staying for months at a time. No two days were alike. Our home pulsated with creative energy, always a meal on the stove that had to be stretched to feed unexpected visitors. That was a usual day. But all of that changed in an instant. For me, for Jessica, for my two sons, and my husband.

After the surgery, we didn't know from one morning to the next if I'd be able to get out of bed. If I could walk, stand, or even sit. If I could make breakfast, lunch, dinner, or those fancy birthday cakes I made before the surgery. They began to realize that I'd never sing, dance, or play music with them again.

I've tried many times to examine how that must've felt to my children. Mothers enter the hospital assuring their young ones they'll return home "better than ever" as the doctor promised, only to leave the hospital to never be the same again.

Sure, our lives had bright moments after the surgery, and they still do. Many beautiful and tender moments. But to say my creative energy and laughter had gone is an understatement. I went from being the center of all the activity, to standing at its edge, doing my best to keep body and soul and family together.

When I say to women, "I know," it's unfortunately because I do. I know all too well what they mean. My work isn't nearly done. I have to find ways to work faster, to be more effective at helping women. Nearly every waking moment, I'm working toward ending the surgical abuse of women. Every minute I lose, another woman's life is destroyed.

FIFTY

Misdiagnosed and mistreated.

Atlanta, Georgia—Nora W. Coffey

Counseling people throughout the last 25 years, I often listen without comment as women occasionally refer to their doctors in racially derogatory ways or defend their actions, saying things like, "But he's a Christian, Nora. If a Christian doctor tells me I need the surgery, then I must need it," as if religious affiliation will protect her and abusive treatment is limited to doctors of different ethnic or cultural backgrounds than her own.

I'm committed to helping women take in complex information, regardless of what other issues are influencing their decision-making process. For a variety of reasons, it sometimes takes a while to determine exactly what happened when, and what details are relevant.

I spoke with a woman a couple of years before the protests who I'll call Claudette. She made an appointment to talk about some problems she was having from a fibroid "as big as a grapefruit." She had such a rich, Southern drawl and her speech was so unusual it was difficult for me to understand what she was saying.

The conversation began with a discussion about uterine artery embolization. Although the fibroid was benign and asymptomatic, the doctor insisted she needed a hysterectomy. "But I didn't want one," she said, so I assumed she had avoided hysterectomy. "I feel fine and weren't in no pain," she said. She switched doctors at her husband's urging, after the doctor who'd recommended hysterectomy rested his hands on her thighs. Claudette then told me she was involved in a class-action lawsuit and that she'd already undergone the UAE. She then ended the conversation by saying she'd had her last "sacka" (which I deduced was her term for menstruation) five months earlier, and that she wanted to be compensated for what the doctors had taken from her. It was only then that I realized she'd been hysterectomized.

In our next call Claudette said she believed the doctor hysterectomized her because he was "a dirty Jew," so she went to another doctor to find out why she was having such a hard time after the surgery. And several more doctors after that. But none of them said her problems were a result of the hysterectomy. She refused to give up, though, and somehow found HERS.

Claudette struggled to control her emotions and groped for the words to explain herself in a tongue that was so unlike my own it was almost like speaking different languages. She wasn't sure herself what happened, and that's why she called HERS. At every turn she apologized for bothering me, for complaining, for swearing, for being a burden to her husband, for being so much trouble to everyone.

Long before the hysterectomy, and prior to the UAE, a doctor recommended an intrauterine device (IUD) known as the Dalkon Shield as a form of contraception. The doctor didn't inform Claudette that IUDs were well known by then to cause severe problems in women and would ultimately result in more than 300,000 lawsuits and billions of dollars of litigation.[183]

An IUD is inserted into the uterus by a doctor, and a string hangs down from the cervix so it can be removed at a later date.

---

[183]   Perry, Susan and Dawson, Jim, *Nightmare: Women and the Dalkon Shield*, Macmillan, 1985. Sovol, Richard B., *Bending The Law: the Story of the Dalkon Shield Bankruptcy*, University of Chicago Press, 1991.

It's normal for there to be bacteria in the vagina, where it remains unless it's pushed into the uterus through the cervix by medical devices, IUDS, or tampons that aren't changed regularly. If a pathway is created, the bacteria that is harmless in the vagina can become an infection in the uterus. It's common for vaginal bacteria to travel up the string into the uterus and fallopian tubes, causing infections and a host of other problems and unnecessary treatments, including foreign-body inflammation/reaction, adhesions, occlusion (blocking) of the fallopian tubes, ectopic pregnancies, birth deformities, sterility, castration, and even death, if the problems go untreated.

Another woman I counseled named Patricia developed sepsis, a life-threatening systemic infection, after using a Dalkon Shield IUD. She was hysterectomized and castrated at the age of 23. She joined the class-action lawsuit against A.H. Robins, the company that marketed the device, and was awarded a mere $750. After the surgery she suffered extreme fatigue, loss of sexual feeling, loss of identity, loss of vitality, joint pain, short-term memory loss, and a host of other common post-hysterectomy and castration problems. She was heroic in continuing with her education, becoming a professor in New York, but her physical problems became progressively unbearable. When she reached a point where she couldn't cope with her problems anymore, this highly intelligent, compassionate, and exotically beautiful woman ended her life.

In Claudette's case, she also began experiencing problems soon after using a Dalkon Shield IUD. She went back to the doctor and an MRI (magnetic resonance imaging) was performed. The MRI clearly showed the presence of Pelvic Inflammatory Disease. She should never have been given an IUD in the first place, but right then and there she should've been treated for PID, and her symptoms and the infection would most likely have resolved. But the doctor neglected to properly culture and treat the infection. Instead he performed a UAE on a woman with PID, which made the infection worse.

She did have fibroids, and one of them was large, but they were asymptomatic and incidental to the real problem, which is that the string on the IUD provided a pathway for pathogens. So a UAE was performed, while the easily diagnosed infection was neglected.

Her problems continued. When she went back to the doctor with the same problems as before the UAE, he insisted that now she needed a hysterectomy. So she was admitted into the hospital under the assumption that a hysterectomy would solve the pelvic pain she was experiencing. Without appropriate treatment of the PID, and without informed consent about the effects of the surgery, Claudette was hysterectomized and castrated.

When she opened her eyes, the first thing she saw was her husband praying over her. He stayed up all night, because he thought she was dying. She stayed in the hospital for a month afterwards, fighting the life-threatening sepsis that had developed from the spreading PID. As she spent the first few months coping with the loss of her female organs, she was also being administered intravenous antibiotics through a PIC Line in her chest. At long last she was getting the treatment she needed to treat the infection, but not before another doctor treated her benign fibroids with a UAE, and not before she was hysterectomized and castrated. It's amazing she survived.

No one bothered to explain any of this to Claudette or her husband. So she sent her records to HERS and asked me to figure out what was done to her. After all of the negligence, lies, and blunders, she finally found out what had been done to her.

In our next conversation Claudette's husband was on the phone with us again. He was having a hard time understanding why Claudette let all of this be done to her. It took him a while to figure out that it wasn't her fault. Claudette made the best decision she could with the information she was provided with by doctors she thought were experts.

The IUD was deemed safe in the early 1970s by Hugh Davis, M.D., a faculty member of the Johns Hopkins Medical School, who was entitled to a percentage of the profits from the Dalkon Shield. He published an article called "The Shield: a Superior Modern Contraceptive" and skewed the results of a very small unscientific study to make the IUD appear to be safe. Then the Dalkon Shield was marketed to the public with lavish advertising campaigns in the years before FDA began testing medical devices. The inventors and the A.H. Robins Company, which bought the rights to it, profited greatly from it, even as it damaged the women who used it. Robins sold the company to American Home Products (now Wyeth), which reportedly made more money from interest on their profits than they paid out in claims from women harmed by their destructive product.[184]

"I don't know how all that was done to me just for an infection," Claudette said, "but I don't think I need another doctor. I need a lawyer." And then it was my job to tell her that she faced an uphill battle finding a doctor to be an expert witness, and that

[184] Ibid.

if she won her case the damages awarded would most likely be limited by so-called "frivolous lawsuit" legislation.

As we were getting set up for the Atlanta protest, some of the other protestors seemed bothered by the husband of a woman I'll call Virginia. They found him controlling and overbearing, so they told him Virginia would be okay at the protest without him. They asked me my opinion whether he should stay or not, but I said nothing. Having counseled her, I sensed there might be more to this picture than the protestors could see at first blush. Her husband gave in, but instead of leaving Virginia alone with us altogether, he parked across street and kept an eye on her from there, which seemed to bother a few of the others.

The Southeast was in the grip of yet another cold snap. There was very little pedestrian traffic, but we began distributing information the best we could. I instinctively kept an eye on Virginia. She walked back and forth on the sidewalk for a while and spoke with a few pedestrians. But then quite unexpectedly, she turned and walked into the street. I was far enough away from her all I could do was helplessly watch as Virginia unsteadily wandered into the oncoming traffic, like she was sleepwalking. Immediately her husband jumped out of the car. Risking his own safety, he rushed to her side with cars bearing down on them. He gently put his arm around her and carefully guided her back to the sidewalk, ignoring the impatient drivers honking at them to hurry out of the street. I think everyone understood why he stayed at Virginia's elbow after that.

No permit was required for the protest, which took place at the Emory Crawford Long Hospital on Pine Street, between Peachtree Street NE and Peachtree Street NW.

"Do you know what the Georgia state tree is?" Rick asked.

"Well, it must be the peach tree," I replied.

"Nope. It's the Live Oak."

Along with Virginia, a biologist, a nurse, a telephone company worker, and a former GM executive joined me. Joan from Detroit was there too, who further cemented her status as our most prolific Protest & Play participant. From her journal, Joan sent this to us:

> A woman I met in the lobby of the hotel named Nina had come from Jupiter, Florida to visit her cancer-stricken father. She had undergone an unnecessary hysterectomy three years ago at the doctor's recommendation. During the operation, while she was unconscious, the doctor persuaded her husband to sign-off on removal of Nina's healthy ovaries too. Later, when she discovered what was done, she was outraged. I gave her a stack of HERS pamphlets, which she said she would be happy to distribute to friends and relatives.

I thought about the husband of the woman from Florida. Like John from the Tennessee chapter, he couldn't have known better. When the doctor came to the waiting room during the hysterectomy claiming he'd have to remove her ovaries to save her life, he thought he was doing the right thing by signing the consent form. He didn't have time to educate himself about the functions of the female organs as his wife lay opened-up on the operating table. He couldn't have known the right questions to ask the doctor. In what was portrayed as an emergency, he wasn't equipped with the information to challenge the doctor's assertion that castration was medically necessary.

All other factors remaining equal, his wife had less than a .01% chance of ever developing ovarian cancer. In other words, she had a 99% chance of *not* developing ovarian cancer, which is listed as a "rare disease" by the Office of Rare Diseases (ORD) of the National Institutes of Health (NIH).[185] But she shouldn't blame herself or her husband. The doctor performing the surgery either knew that what he was doing wasn't medically necessary and chose to do it anyway or he was ignorant of the anatomical and medical facts and should never have been given a medical degree in the first place. Neither of these reasons is acceptable.

Because Rick's time was divided between the protests and getting the full production of *un becoming* on track in Washington, D.C., he wasn't able to protest with us in Georgia. But he was able to organize the reading in Atlanta and oversee one rehearsal before the performance Saturday afternoon at the Wyndham Atlanta Hotel.

Cynthia, a drama teacher from Spelman College, supplied the *un becoming* cast in Atlanta with music stands. I had counseled her for fibroids after a doctor told her the only treatment option for her "condition" was hysterectomy. She was alarmed to learn in one brief phone call with me what the doctor neglected to inform her of in multiple medical consultations. She was stunned at the enormity of the problem of hysterectomy and the way that her experience with doctors was so accurately reflected in Rick's play. It's enough to make you wonder if doctors aren't more likely to hysterectomize vibrant, intelligent, and attractive women…to take away from them something they can't have or be themselves.

Cynthia brought her teenage daughter and a few students to the fine reading of *un becoming* by VisionQuest Theater Company. In the talkback she told us, "I'm forever grateful to HERS."

---

[185] http://www.wrongdiagnosis.com/o/ovarian_cancer/prevalence.htm.

It was her birthday, and she asked her daughter to attend the play with her as a birthday gift.

The next day, because Emory Crawford Long was set back from the street, the other protestors who lived in Atlanta wanted to try a different hospital. So we switched locations. Once we got there I got a call from Cynthia, asking, "I'm here at the hospital, where are you guys?" Because of the cold rain, she had brought along enough umbrellas for all of us.

Each protest was like a refuge. It was a supportive environment where we could speak freely about how hysterectomy had changed our lives. It was comforting to once again realize that people of disparate backgrounds could be brought together by a common cause that transcended our differences. Disparities weren't important once we were united by the common cause of doing everything we could to stop hysterectomy from becoming the legacy of another generation of girls. We listened to each other's experiences with understanding and empathy. We agreed to continue working together to change the law. And when I look at the protest photos it's very clear—the support, attention, and determination is obvious on our faces.

FIFTY-ONE

It's not nice to complain.

Charleston, South Carolina—Nora W. Coffey

Once I arrived in Charleston, no map was required. All I had to do was follow the towering construction crane to the Medical University of South Carolina Hospital (MUSC). The $275M expansion project added nine operating rooms and 156 hospital rooms.[186] And that was only Phase I of the massive project. That may seem like a lot of money, but I've been told that most operating rooms average more than 1,000 surgeries each year. Since the average cost of a hysterectomy in the U.S. is about $25,000,[187] those nine operating rooms alone could generate as much revenue in one year as the total cost of this expansion project. For the fiscal year ending June 30, 2007, MUSC reported revenue of $1.5B.[188]

The parking lots nearest to the hospital were so overrun with construction equipment I had to park a few blocks away. There wasn't anywhere to stockpile materials and foot traffic was so heavy, I had to make repeated trips to get more.

As I walked back and forth between the hospital and the rental car, it struck me more in Charleston than in any other city that America is becoming a society of contrasts. I parked the rental car around the corner, on an affluent street with high-end shops.

---

[186] "NBBJ Designs $275m S.C. Medical Center," *Real Estate Weekly*, February 27, 2008.
[187] HERS Foundation. Conservative estimate of immediate hospital and doctor-related charges. Does not include additional costs incurred for treatment of chronic adverse effects of the surgery.
[188] MUSC 2006-2007 Annual Report, http://www.musc.edu/pr/annual_report.pdf.

The well put-together boutique shoppers didn't seem to have a care in the world. But back at the protest site, one woman after another told me she was unable to maintain her previous level of employment after hysterectomy. And I can't remember any other city where so many women told me they were afraid their husbands were about to leave them because they had so many health problems and didn't enjoy sex after the surgery.

Each time I ran out of pamphlets it was like stepping through an invisible wall out of reality and into a world of privilege and ease. As they passed from one shop to the next, a few of the trendy women I gave pamphlets to as I headed back to the protest seemed disgusted by the information. Clearly hysterectomy was just as much of a problem there as it was around the corner, but the shoppers preferred that hysterectomy not be spoken about. It was an oddly fitting end to the protest year to be a witness to both worlds by simply turning a corner.

Charleston is a charming city with a mild climate, but the southern hospitality and gentility don't hide what's being done to women there. Educating women in the South is particularly difficult because of the culture of pleasantry. It's not polite for women to question doctors there. And it's certainly not acceptable to talk about private matters like sexuality in public.

As we traveled across the country to protest against unconsented hysterectomy, we learned a lot about who we are as Americans. And we learned a lot about the importance of geography and regional culture on the landscape of our experiences. Women in the South are 50% more likely to be hysterectomized than women in the Northeast, and black women are 20% more likely to be hysterectomized than white women.[189] All women are vulnerable, but a black woman in the South is at a much higher risk than a white woman in the Northeast.

And I learned a lot about myself too. The women's voices I knew so well from counseling them over the phone now had faces. What I didn't anticipate is how much more I'd absorb their pain and anguish. I carried their wounded spirits with me from one city to the next. So even at the protests where no one joined me, I never felt truly alone. My voice was their voice.

Rick and I truly lacked a map and a compass. Long before we met each other, we both attended and led other protests, but nothing else compared to the Protest & Play year. As Alfred Korzybski said, "A map is not the territory."[190]

Similarly, anatomical drawings of the female pelvis give us a visual rendering of the pelvic organs and how they're attached in the pelvis, but they're as inadequate when describing female anatomy as a road atlas is in describing the people of South Carolina.

Anatomical drawings fail to reveal the void left inside a woman's pelvis when the uterus is severed from its attachments and removed. They fail to reveal how, when a woman stands after surgery, the void causes other organs to drift and rest unnaturally against other organs and tissues they once buttressed. They fail to reveal how the flow of blood throughout the pelvis, genitalia, legs, and feet is compromised by hysterectomy. They fail to reveal the ways that structural integrity in the pelvis is destroyed, or how

---

[189]   Centers for Disease Control and Prevention (CDC), National Center for Health Statistics (NCHS).
[190]   Korzybski, Alfred, "A Non-Aristotelian System and its Necessity for Rigour in Mathematics and Physics," a paper presented before the American Mathematical Society, New Orleans, December 28, 1931.

severing the nerves will cause a loss of sensation throughout a woman's body. No matter how detailed the drawing may be, the far-reaching impact of what's done to women, their families, their friends, and society as a whole cannot be completely conveyed by a drawing.

When so many women are as eager for information as they were in South Carolina, it's difficult deciding precisely which moment to stop protesting. But at about 1:00 p.m. on Sunday I had once again run out of pamphlets and it was time to go. I had planned to only protest on Saturday. But after flying back to Washington, D.C. on Saturday to take care of a few matters, I got back on a plane Sunday morning to protest another day in Charleston.

As I boarded the plane back to Washington I was eager to get the D.C. events underway, but one foot was reluctant to leave South Carolina. Like Mississippi, I could've spent many weeks there and still never scratched the surface of the desperate need for information that doctors and hospitals deny women.

As the plane lifted up into the clouds, I tried to nap. But when I closed my eyes I couldn't get an image from the protest out of my head. It was of a young woman walking slowly toward me in Charleston. When she finally stood at my side, she said only, "It was done to me right here," pointing toward the Medical University of South Carolina Hospital. She had long, light-brown hair, green eyes, and freckles. She was only 20 years old, but she needed a cane to walk. I handed her a pamphlet and she eagerly read it. We talked for a while, and then she tucked the pamphlet into her purse and said, "Well, I came all this way to say thanks for what you're doing." She then turned and limped away.

FIFTY-TWO

From revolution to resolution.

Washington, DC—Rick Schweikert

The Protest & Play year will someday be recognized as one of the cornerstones of the foundation for legislative change to end the worst medical atrocity of all time. It represents the need for action and the public's desire to let the world know that not only does hysterectomy damage individuals, it damages families and society as a whole.

For every person who joined us, there were many thousands more who were committed to doing what they could, even if they were unable to be there with us. Many said they'd change their party vote for a legislator, governor, or president for a candidate who was committed to shepherding a hysterectomy consent law that includes the HERS anatomy video through the legislative process. Most weren't able to stand on a street wearing the equivalent of a scarlet H in front of an unwelcoming hospital, but they are able to pull a lever for a politician who will stop this madness from damaging future generations.

Women who may have little in common prior to the surgery have everything in common after. But until HERS was formed, they lacked organization, a common goal, and a figurehead to create lasting change. The Protest & Play year established HERS as the central organization of a powerful, single-issue entity.

Their demand was clear—gynecologists must be prevented from hysterectomizing another generation of women. The potential membership was massive—more than 22 million hysterectomized women alive today (along with their friends and family) in every corner of the country. And now HERS was helping them organize as a powerful political influence.

Strapping an uninformed woman to a gurney and removing her female organs should be considered unlawful detention by the justice system. In any other arena than a hospital operating room, the perpetrator would be locked away from society for such violent behavior. It's women who're getting the life sentences, when it's the doctors who deserve punishment for denying women their right to informed consent.

Our final protest would take place in the city where the legislators who represent us vote yea or nay to the laws that regulate the behavior of a nation. In the absence of a law mandating hysterectomy informed consent, the hysterectomy rate continues to rise. Throughout this book we have said that "at least" 621,000 women are hysterectomized each year. Although government reports indicate that the rate has remained steady, the hysterectomy rate is actually increasing. As Nora says, "The number of hysterectomies being performed on women is *grossly* underreported and could be well over a million each year."

The reason for this discrepancy in the numbers is that hysterectomies performed in hospitals and surgical centers funded by the federal government aren't included in the NCHS data. The large number of women counseled by HERS over the years who were hysterectomized in military and Indian reservation hospitals is a clear indication of how large a number that might be. Other hysterectomies that aren't reported in the Hospital Discharge Survey (from which the NCHS derives its statistics) include hysterectomies performed outside the country (a practice dubbed "medical tourism"[191]) and

---

[191] Surgeries performed on U.S. citizens in foreign countries are projected to top six million each year, according to "Explosive Growth in Medical Tourism and Rise of Retail Clinics Provide Huge Cost Savings for Patients," *Deloitte Center for Health Solutions*, July 30, 2008.

hysterectomies performed in outpatient surgical centers and hospitals where women are discharged in less than 24 hours.

Outpatient hysterectomy is as invisible to the public eye as the organs removed during the surgery. The assembly-line hysterectomy era has arrived. Women are admitted, hysterectomized, and then pushed back out the door in a matter of hours, without any mention of the lifelong, life-altering consequences of removing the female organs. To get a sense of just how many outpatient hysterectomies are being performed, you don't have to look far. In 2004, *OB/GYN News* reported that 30 percent of hysterectomized women in an 18-month study were sent home after 12 hours. Other studies demonstrate a similar trend.[192]

Furthermore, a study published in the *American Journal of Public Health* found that "more women reported hysterectomy

---

[192]   Boschert, Sherry, "Early discharge OK in laparoscopic hysterectomy: avoiding an overnight stay." *OB/GYN News*, Feb 1, 2004. See also Pollard, R. and Ahluwalia, P. "Safety and Patient Satisfaction of Outpatient Total Laparoscopic Hysterectomy," *Journal of Minimally Invasive Gynecology*, Volume 12, Issue 5, Page 19. One of the conclusions is that "patients will be satisfied with same day discharge." See also Levy, B. et al., "Outpatient vaginal hysterectomy is safe for patients and reduces institutional cost," *Journal of Minimally Invasive Gynecology*, Volume 12, Issue 6, pp. 494-501, in which the authors claim "same-day discharge after vaginal hysterectomy is safe and feasible in the vast majority of patients." Powers, Thomas W. et al., "The Outpatient Vaginal Hysterectomy," *American Journal of Obstetrics & Gynecology*, 168(6):1875-1880, June 1993: "This small pilot study adds to the growing body of literature that demonstrates the safety and feasibility of performing vaginal hysterectomy." Hoffman, C. P. et al., "Laparoscopic hysterectomy: the Kaiser Permanente San Diego experience," *Journal of Minimally Invasive Gynecology* 2005 Jan-Feb: "Same-day discharge for LSH occurred in 25.1% of patients." Penketh, R. et al., "A Prospective Observational Study of the Safety and Acceptability of Vaginal Hysterectomy Performed in a 24-Hour Day Case Surgery Setting," *Obstetrical & Gynecological Survey*, July 2007: "Opening of an ambulatory care unit provided an opportunity to evaluate vaginal hysterectomy when performed in a 24-hour day case surgery setting with follow-up telephone support....More than 90% of women were discharged home within 24 hours of surgery."

than could be confirmed by hospital records."[193] As a matter of fact, more than 33% of the women studied said they had been hysterectomized, but no hospital verification could be found. It's difficult to imagine a woman claiming to have been hysterectomized, unless she had. Maybe a more accurate interpretation of these findings would be, "One third of all hysterectomies aren't reported by hospitals."

This hidden population means that far more than one out of three women under 60 in the U.S. has been hysterectomized. The real number might be closer to one in two. Living in the Northeast, it might not seem possible, but after traveling across the South and Midwest, where we met as many women who were hysterectomized as not, it seems more than possible. In Mississippi it appears to be quite probable.

Gynecology is altering the very way we define "woman." When you consider what it is to be a woman of 60 versus what it is to be a man of 60, consider the fact that as many as half of those women have had their sex organs removed while almost none of the men have.

The silent epidemic of hysterectomy lurks in every corner. In each city we visited, all we had to do was say the H word and people stepped out of the shadows to speak openly about their experiences.

Nora caught a taxi at the Washington National Airport, and the driver asked her why she was in town. When Nora told him about the HERS conference and the protest on Capitol Hill, he

---

[193] Brett, Kate and Madans, Jennifer, "Hysterectomy Use: The Correspondence Between Self-Reports and Hospital Records, *American Journal of Public Health*, October 1994.

began talking about the problems his wife was having since a doctor hysterectomized her. "She's only 35," he said, "and she can't stop crying." She underwent a hysterectomy about three years before, he said, and it left her partially disabled, with chronic fibromyalgia (widespread joint and muscle pain) and debilitating back pain.

As Nora made her way back to Washington from her second trip to Charlotte, I was struggling to salvage a production of *un becoming*. Things hadn't gone as planned, and I was preoccupied with doing everything I could to make sure the play hit the mark at the Warehouse Theater. The play couldn't have been staged in a more ideal venue, but the theater company we hired was woefully unprepared for the task of producing it. Remarkably, the cast did a good job, in spite of the director, and audiences responded to it. After one of the performances, a woman pulled me aside. She gestured to the man standing behind her, and whispered, "Maybe now he'll understand a little better what I've been going through."

The play opened on March 3rd, the protests began with a march on Capitol Hill on March 11th, and the conference was held on Saturday, March 12th. It was inevitable that the police would show up at the Capitol Hill protest, so I wasn't surprised when someone came for me, saying, "They have a problem with our protest boundaries." The issue was that we were resting some of our protest signs against public property. "We're the public," I told the officer, "and that *is* public property."

"Either you move them or we will," he said.

Later a few more cops stopped by to tell us we could only protest in and around the park and not on the sidewalk across the street. When I asked why, they said, "Because you're obstructing pedestrians."

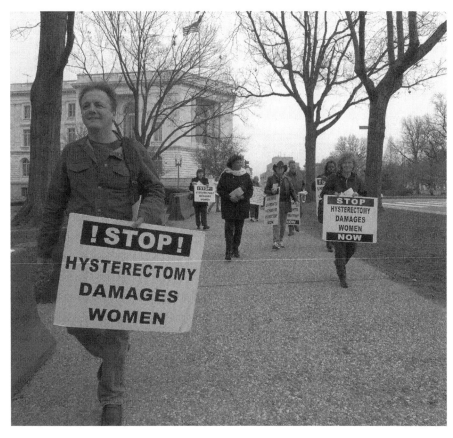

The next time the police arrived (the third time in just the first hour) they told us we couldn't protest on *any* of the sidewalks except for the ones inside the park. "Your demonstration is confined to the interior of the park," he said, "or we're going to shut you down." Our permit clearly included the public sidewalks in and around the park, so I called the officer who issued the permit to us and told her what was going on. She said, "No, don't worry. He's wrong. You have every right to be there. I'll jump in my car and come down." Just a few minutes later she arrived, telling the other officer we were in the right and had a legal permit. When she left she took a handful of pamphlets to give to her co-workers in the permit office. As she got into her car she said she'd try to make it to one of the last performances of *un becoming*.

Some of the protestors stood talking in groups, while others marched around and through Upper Senate Park. A uniformed security guard with a wire to his ear approached Nora. He told her we weren't allowed to protest on the sidewalks inside the park. Nora laughed, asking him why, since we had a permit to do exactly that. He repeated what the cops had said—"Because you're obstructing pedestrians." No one had obstructed any pedestrians, and we weren't about to be denied our rights in the nation's capital, so we ignored him and he went away.

At some point a protestor spotted a reporter from CNN. Thinking he was there to report on the protest, we were disappointed when he told Nora he had just finished interviewing a politician. The reporter was initially dismissive, but Nora surprised him by saying, "This is more important than your next appointment."

He paused from packing up his equipment. "Really...?"

"This is about *your* life," Nora said, "not just the lives of the women and men and children who are out here protesting with us today. It's about everyone you care about, because every woman, man, and child you know can be affected by this."

Most Capitol Hill protests he'd seen were obnoxious, with megaphones and repetitive chants. In a city accustomed to tuning them out, he said it was refreshing to see a different kind of protest.

Nora quickly laid out why hysterectomy consent was an important issue. He seemed absorbed by what she was saying, but he said he didn't have any control over getting media out there to give us coverage. "We don't have much say anymore about what we report on," he said. Many journalists like him, he said, were muzzled by the politicians they were assigned to. What he could and couldn't write about was decided by editors who were constantly hounded by politicians—the endless back-and-forth between politics and the fourth estate, which former Bush press secretary Scott McClellan calls "the permanent campaign."[194] The reporter said his stories were usually edited down to diluted, "politically-corrected" versions of what he handed in. He resumed packing up his equipment, and then he asked Nora to take a walk down the sidewalk away from the crowd of gathering protestors.

"There are things going on in the House right now that you should know about," he said.

Nora was surprised by his sudden change of tone and body language. "I'm not aware of anything going on in Congress about hysterectomy," Nora replied. "Tell me."

"Well…I can't," he said.

"Why not?"

"I just can't."

"You mean you can, but you choose not to…."

"No, I mean I can't. I'm not supposed to know. It's really important though, so you've got to find out about this."

He gave Nora the contact information of a colleague who he said would be able to talk about it. Nora called them and left a voicemail, but she didn't get a return call. We searched the internet and made a few calls, but we never heard any news about anything that happened on Capitol Hill about hysterectomy that entire month. Whatever he was referring to remains a mystery.

[194]   McClellan, Scott, *What Happened*, PublicAffairs, 2008.

Another Capitol Hill reporter said, "I know everything you're saying is true, and some Senators inside these buildings know it's true. But I also know they don't care." He paused to scan the disappointed faces of the protestors gathering around. Then he said, "And they're never going to care." And then, after another pause, he said, "They're never going to change." And with that he crossed the street and entered the Capitol Building.

The other protestors were stunned. I think it was probably the first time they realized that the problem of hysterectomy is more than just a matter of education. Nora said to the protestors, "For many people it's known, but it's politically unfavorable to point a finger at doctors and corporate medicine." The recognition that Nora was right began to register on their faces. Before walking away Nora said, "But they have changed in the past. The power of our votes will make them change again. It's important to talk about the issues, to be public, to make the statement that this matters in every state, but we'll have to do more than talk about the issues to change things in a lasting way. We're sowing the seeds for change. We've counseled women in every corner of the country, but now we're organizing in every state. Next we'll use the courts and the government to act on our behalf," she said, "as they're directed by the Constitution. Politicians need to know that if they want to remain our elected officials, they'll have to represent us, not the medical industry. The vote is mightier than medical industry dollars," she said. "There's a whole lot of apathy in this country about politics and the feeling that votes don't matter. But people are willing to vote on this single issue."

One of the protestors spotted Senator Kennedy's limousine. It caused quite a stir when Ellen ran up to his car and the Senator put his window down to take a pamphlet. He and Ellen had a brief exchange, and then he drove away.

The only other politician to stop by spoke with a protestor who was a nurse and teacher who later provided this journal entry:

> Washington, DC was clearly a different arena compared to the other protests I attended. We protested outside the capital building. One senator told me point blank that he knows now that he lost his wife through divorce as a direct consequence following the aftermath of her hysterectomy. He told me he would take additional literature inside and to keep up the good work. Of course there were also those who felt they didn't need the information. I had a student with me. He got tired of the rejection so he decided to leave information on cars. He never expected such rejection in trying to educate the public.

For four days following the Capitol Hill protest, we were in front of George Washington University Hospital. We distributed thousands of pamphlets near a Metro station.

One doctor yelled at me, "Hysterectomy is not castration!" although I said nothing of the sort. A student walking by asked, "What's his problem? The teachers here are jerks. I'm serious. I can't stand medical school. I thought it would be better here than where I was, but it's worse. A bunch of pretentious jerks. Anyway, what's this all about?" We talked for a while, and then she said, "Excellent! Good stuff. Give me a few and I'll slip them around inside the hospital. Keep up the good work!" and she walked away reading the pamphlet.

Nora was pleased with the turnout on Capitol Hill and at George Washington. "This is the first time these protestors have been given a platform to have a voice," Nora said. "It's the first time that we're bigger than our numbers. It can become exponential from here."

There was a camaraderie of supporters who believed that together we could and would end this violence against women. This feeling of mutual support was more obvious than ever at the HERS conference that week. I thought about how Congress traveled to Washington from all 50 states to represent their constituents back home, in the same way that women and men from all over the country had traveled to join us at the HERS conference in our nation's capital.

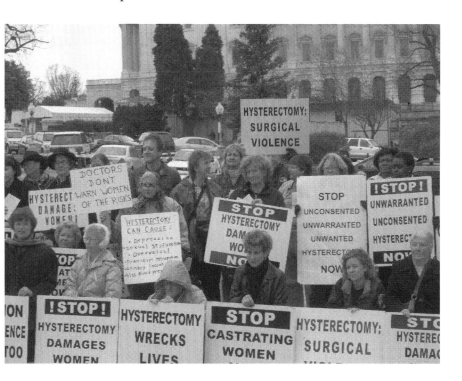

A lasting image from Washington comes to me from a woman I met at one of the performances of *un becoming* at the Warehouse Theater. She arrived with her husband and cried through most of the performance. With tears streaming down her face in the talkback, she told us all the ways that the play matched her own experiences, while her husband sat silently at her side.

After that final performance, we returned to the hotel. There was quite a scene in the hotel lobby with all the long goodbyes. The same woman who spoke up during the talkback was there in the lobby too, waiting for the airport shuttle with her husband.

When Nora passed by the couple, the woman pulled Nora aside to tell her how much the conference and play meant to her, as her husband stood there staring down at his shoes. After Nora said goodbye to her, we returned to our rooms to wash up before we headed out for lunch.

When we met in the lobby about an hour later, we were surprised to see the woman walking back into the hotel with her luggage in tow—alone. When she saw Nora she broke down crying again. She was about three times Nora's size, so Nora disappeared in her arms when they hugged, the woman's body heaving with sobs. "I'm just so glad I met you all," she said. "My husband and I got all the way to the airport and I realized he still hadn't said one word to me about any of this. It's just like back home. Since the surgery, no one will talk with me about it. I just can't take it anymore. I knew if I went home he'd never be able to talk about it, and that's just the way we'd live the rest of our lives, but I need to. I need to be around other women who don't mind talking about it. I can't go back there. I can't go back to being silent."

Nora led her over to an area of the lobby with sofas where a group of protestors had gathered. They made space so Nora and the woman could sit down. Grace put an arm around her, Joan took her hand, Mary and Julia stood behind her with a hand on her shoulders, and this time there were no tears. She knew she could talk about everything now. She knew she'd never whisper the H word again and that she was with others who were through being silenced.

Her husband continued home without her. Eventually, she went home too, and a few months later she called Nora to say that her husband did finally break the silence.

What started out as an ancient physician's effort to save the life of a woman with a gangrenous uterus has evolved into the sanctioned mutilation of untold millions of women. Robotic machines now enable surgeons to remove the uterus without getting blood on their hands. As a nation, we're in dire need of legislation to put an end to the barbaric practice of unconsented hysterectomy.

This book portrays a complex problem with a surprisingly simple solution. By giving women the HERS video "Female Anatomy: the Functions of the Female Organs" prior to telling them to sign a hysterectomy consent form, physicians would finally provide women with the information they need to make informed decisions.

Our future is shaped by our actions. The actions of protestors across the country helped educate tens of thousands of people throughout the Protest & Play year. The actions of millions of Americans will be required to stop hysterectomy from becoming the legacy of another generation of girls.

Every day for a year we lived and breathed the tragic stories of medical abuse against women. It was a journey of many thousands of miles, begun with a single step in Birmingham, Alabama. By the end of the protest and play year, we knew hysterectomy and female castration were everywhere in America. In small towns and big cities, on military bases and Native American reservations, in trailer parks and posh resorts. Like a contagious disease, nearly everywhere we visited was distorted by disability, distrust, and the disintegration of women and families.

There is no escaping it. There is only ending it.

END

INDEX